THE SOCIETY FOR APPLIED BACT.
TECHNICAL SERIES NO. 24

Immunological Techniques in Microbiology

Edited by

J.M. GRANGE
Cardiothoracic Institute
University of London
London, U.K.

A. FOX & N.L. MORGAN
South Bank Polytechnic
London, U.K.

BLACKWELL SCIENTIFIC PUBLICATIONS

OXFORD LONDON EDINBURGH

BOSTON PALO ALTO MELBOURNE

© 1987 by the Society for
Applied Bacteriology and published for them by
Blackwell Scientific Publications
Editorial offices:
Osney Mead, Oxford OX2 0EL
(Orders: Tel. 0865 240201)
8 John Street, London WC1N 2ES
23 Ainslie Place, Edinburgh EH3 6AJ
52 Beacon Street, Boston
  Massachusetts 02108, USA
667 Lytton Avenue, Palo Alto
  California 94301, USA
107 Barry Street, Carlton
  Victoria 3053, Australia

First published 1987

Typeset, printed and bound in Great Britain by
William Clowes Limited, Beccles and London

DISTRIBUTORS

USA and Canada
  Blackwell Scientific Publications Inc
  P O Box 50009, Palo Alto
  California 94303
  (Orders: Tel. (415) 965-4081)

Australia
  Blackwell Scientific Publications
  (Australia) Pty Ltd
  107 Barry Street
  Carlton, Victoria 3053
  (Orders: Tel. (03) 347-0300)

British Library
Cataloguing in Publication Data

Immunological techniques in microbiology.
  —(The Society for Applied Bacteriology
  technical series, ISSN 0583-8924; v. 24).
  1. Microbiology—Technique
  2. Immunology
  I. Grange, John M.   II. Fox, Arnold
  III. Morgan, N. L.   IV. Series
  576   QR186

ISBN 0-632-01908-5

Library of Congress
Cataloging-in-Publication Data

Immunological techniques in microbiology.
  (The Society for Applied Bacteriology
  technical series; no. 24).
  Based on the Society for Applied Bacteriology
  Autumn Demonstration Meeting held at the
  South Bank Polytechnic, London, on Oct. 15th,
  1986.
  1. Immunology—Technique—Congresses. 2.
  Antibodies, Monoclonal—Diagnostic use—
  Congresses. 3. Enzyme-linked immunosorbent
  assay—Congresses. 4. Microbiology—
  Technique—Congresses. I. Grange, John M. II.
  Fox, A. (Arnold), 1927–   . III. Morgan, N. L.
  (Neil L.), 1951–   . IV. Society for Applied
  Bacteriology. Demonstration Meeting (1986:
  South Bank Polytechnic). V. Series: Technical
  series (Society for Applied Bacteriology); no. 24.
  [DNLM: 1. Immunologic Technics—congresses.
  2. Microbiology—methods—congresses. WI
  SO851F no. 24/QW 525 I3248 1986].
  QR187.A1I46   1987   576′.028   87-
  21800
  ISBN 0-632-01908-5

Contents

Contributors

C. J. ALBERT, *Department of Biotechnology, South Bank Polytechnic, Borough Road, London SE1 0AA*

S. J. ALCOCK, *Microbiology Department, Campden Food Preservation Research Association, Chipping Campden, Gloucestershire GL55 6LD*

A. ANDERSON, *Syva U.K., St. Ives House, Maidenhead, Berks SL6 1QS*

P. T. ATKEY, *Glasshouse Crops Research Institute, Worthing Road, Littlehampton, West Sussex BN17 6LP*

P. K. C. AUSTWICK, *Robens Institute of Industrial and Environmental Health and Safety, University of Surrey, Guildford, Surrey GU2 5HX*

J. S. BECK, *Department of Pathology, Ninewells Hospital and Medical School, The University, Dundee DD1 9SY*

P. R. BERRY, *Food Hygiene Laboratory, Central Public Health Laboratory, 61 Colindale Avenue, London NW9 5HT*

J. F. CHAUVEAU, *Service de la Protection des Végétaux, Angers, France*

J. A. CLAYDEN, *Microbiology Department, Campden Food Preservation Research Association, Chipping Campden, Gloucestershire GL55 6LD*

G. COGHILL, *Department of Pathology, Ninewells Hospital and Medical School, The University, Dundee DD1 9SY*

P. COOK, *City of London Polytechnic, Department of Biological Sciences, Old Castle Street, London E1 7NT*

J. H. CREEDY, *LKB Instruments Ltd, 232 Addington Road, Selsdon, Surrey CR2 8YD*

R. J. S. DUNCAN, *Wellcome Diagnostics, Langley Court, Beckenham, Kent BR3 3BS*

R. S. FAWKES, *Department of Pathology, Ninewells Hospital and Medical School, The University, Dundee DD1 9SY*

C. R. FRICKER, *Department of Microbiology, University of Reading, London Road, Reading RG1 5AQ*

C. GAYLARDE, *City of London Polytechnic, Department of Biological Sciences, Old Castle Street, London E1 7NT*

J. H. GIBBS, *Department of Pathology, Ninewells Hospital and Medical School, The University, Dundee DD1 9SY*

P. A. GIBBS, *Leatherhead Food Research Association, Randalls Road, Leatherhead, Surrey KT22 7RY*

J. A. GIBSON, *Department of Microbiology, Cardiothoracic Institute, Brompton Hospital, Fulham Road, London SW3 6HP*

R. J. GILBERT, *Food Hygiene Laboratory, Central Public Health Laboratory, 61 Colindale Avenue, London NW9 5HT*

S. G. HADFIELD, *Wellcome Research Laboratories, Langley Court, Beckenham, Kent BR3 3BS*

S. D. HAINES, *Leatherhead Food Research Association, Randalls Road, Leatherhead, Surrey KT22 7RY*

P. S. JACKETT, *MRC Tuberculosis and Related Infections Unit, Hammersmith Hospital, Ducane Road, London W12 0HS*

J. D. JANSE, *Plant Protection Service, Wageningen, The Netherlands.*

N. F. JOUY, *Wellcome Research Laboratories, Langley Court, Beckenham, Kent BR3 3BS*

D. M. KEMENY, *Department of Medicine, United Medical and Dental Schools, Guy's Hospital, St. Thomas' Street, London SE1 9RT*

R. LAKE, *Immunology Section, Department of Biophysics, Cell and Molecular Biology, King's College, Manresa Road, London SW3 6LX*

J. L. LONGBOTTOM, *Department of Allergy and Clinical Immunology, Cardiothoracic Institute, Brompton Hospital, Fulham Road, London SW3 6HP*

M. B. MCILLMURRAY, *Wellcome Research Laboratories, Langley Court, Beckenham, Kent BR3 3BS*

M. F. MCINTYRE, *Public Health Laboratory, Dulwich Hospital, East Dulwich Grove, London SE22 8QF*

A. MORGAN, *Immunology Section, Department of Biophysics, Cell and Molecular Biology, King's College, Manresa Road, London SW3 6LX*

N. L. MORGAN, *Department of Biotechnology, South Bank Polytechnic, Borough Road, London SE1 0AA*

R. W. A. PARK, *Department of Microbiology, University of Reading, London Road, Reading, RG1 5AQ*

P. D. PATEL, *Leatherhead Food Research Association, Randalls Road, Leatherhead, Surrey KT22 7RY*

J. PELLY, *Sera-Lab Ltd, Crawley Down, West Sussex RH10 4FF*

J. A. PRICE, *Department of Allergy and Clinical Immunology, Cardiothoracic Institute, Brompton Hospital, Fulham Road, London SW3 6HP*

D. RICHARDS, *Department of Medicine, United Medical and Dental Schools, Guy's Hospital, St. Thomas' Street, London SE1 9RT*

J. C. RODHOUSE, *Food Hygiene Laboratory, Central Public Health Laboratory, 61 Colindale Avenue, London NW9 5HT*

M. A. RUISSEN, *Department of Phytopathology, Agricultural University, Wageningen, The Netherlands*

M. G. SMITH, *Microbiology Department, Kingston Hospital, Galsworthy Road, Kingston Upon Thames, Surrey KT2 7BG*

K. SPEARS, *Department of Biotechnology, South Bank Polytechnic, Borough Road, London SE1 0AA*

N. STAINES, *Immunology Section, Department of Biophysics, Cell and Molecular Biology, King's College, Manresa Road, London SW3 6LX*

C. J. STANNARD, *Leatherhead Food Research Association, Randalls Road, Leatherhead, Surrey KT22 7RY*

D. E. STEAD, *Ministry of Agriculture, Fisheries and Food, Harpenden Laboratory, Hatching Green, Harpenden, Herts AL5 2BD*

M. F. STRINGER, *Microbiology Department, Campden Food Preservation Research Association, Chipping Campden, Gloucestershire GL55 6LD*

M. L. TAYLOR, *Department of Allergy and Clinical Immunology, Cardiothoracic Institute, Brompton Hospital, Fulham Road, London SW3 6HP*

R. W. TINDLE, *Sera-Lab Ltd, Crawley Down, West Sussex RH10 4FF*

J. VAN VAERENBERGH, *Research Institute for Plant Pathology, Merelbeke, Belgium*

J. W. L. VAN VUURDE, *Research Institute for Plant Protection, Wageningen, The Netherlands*

A. A. WIENEKE, *Food Hygiene Laboratory, Central Public Health Laboratory, 61 Colindale Avenue, London NW9 5HT*

D. A. WOOD, *Glasshouse Crops Research Institute, Worthing Road, Littlehampton, West Sussex BN17 6LP*

Preface

In recent years there have been many technical developments in immunology that have potential or actual applications in many other branches of the life sciences. These developments include a number of ultrasensitive systems for the detection and assay of a wide range of biological materials including micro-organisms and their products as well as techniques for isolating and purifying micro-organisms and other antigenic materials. Two developments in particular have greatly extended the scope and applicability of immunological methods; namely the production of monoclonal antibodies and the introduction of enzyme linked immunoassay as a simple, safe and economical alternative to radioimmunoassay.

Although originating from the discipline of immunology, many of the methods require little or no knowledge of, or experience in, that discipline and their ever-growing application is greatly facilitated by automation and by the increasing number of commercially available self-contained kits.

The purpose of this edition of the Society for Applied Bacteriology Technical Series is to describe a number of the currently available techniques and to illustrate how they have been successfully utilized by workers in many branches of microbiology.

This book is based on the Society for Applied Bacteriology Autumn Demonstration Meeting held at the South Bank Polytechnic, London, on 15 October 1986. The editors wish to thank all the contributors for the time and effort they devoted to the demonstration meeting and to the preparation of their manuscripts. We also thank the staff of the Department of Biotechnology of the South Bank Polytechnic for their help in arranging the demonstration meeting.

J. M. Grange
A. Fox
N. L. Morgan

Production of Monoclonal Antibodies

RICHARD LAKE, ADRIENNE MORGAN AND NORMAN STAINES
Immunology Section, Department of Biophysics, Cell and Molecular Biology, King's College, Manresa Road, London SW3 6LX

Introduction

Monoclonal antibodies (MAbs) are valuable to microbiologists because of their great potential as standardized serological reagents for use in the identification and isolation of micro-organisms. It is also clear that such reagents are potentially valuable in both therapy and prophylaxis. These antibodies are the products of individual clones of lymphocytes and are powerful immunologically specific reagents and analytical probes. Because of its homogeneity each MAb can be precisely defined in terms of its specificity and affinity, it is of one immunoglobulin (Ig) class, and can be prepared in large amounts. The methodology involved in the production of MAbs enables the derivation of specific antibodies from animals immunized with impure antigens.

This paper describes the technology that has been developed to prepare MAbs of pre-selected specificity, which can be broadly divided into three steps: first, the fusion of lymphocytes with myeloma cells to make somatic cell hybrids which secrete a specific antibody; second, the separation of different hybrid cells from each other and, third, the propagation of them as cell lines, each making one antibody. The production of MAbs is crucially dependent upon the availability of tissue culture facilities. With this investment and the involvement of experienced workers it will still take several months to isolate stable cloned cell lines producing MAbs in even the simplest system. The amount of long-term tissue culture involved is such that the culture facility must be maintained reliably and be available continuously. There is no doubt that the most efficient way to produce MAbs is to dedicate a facility to doing nothing else. In this way the needs of several research groups might be met by one culture laboratory.

It is not our intention to describe standard tissue culture procedures in detail, but the following items, likely to be readily available in microbiology laboratories, are essential.

Immunological Techniques
in Microbiology

1 A tissue culture hood: a vertical laminar air flow cabinet is ideal.
2 An incubator that can be maintained at 37 °C with a humidified (saturated) atmosphere of 5% CO_2 in air.
3 A liquid nitrogen storage and freezing facility for cell lines.
4 Inverted phase contrast microscope.
5 Bench top centrifuge.
6 Other supporting facilities for tissue culture work including sterilizing oven, refrigerator, autoclave and deep freeze.

General Principles for Producing MAbs

B-lymphocytes that secrete antibodies will not survive *in vitro* beyond a few days or at best a few weeks. Thus, the immortalization of B-cells in a way in which they continue to secrete specific antibodies is the key step in producing MAbs. It must be said at this stage that there are many methods that differ only in detail: we will describe the methods used successfully in our laboratory to prepare DNA-reactive monoclonal autoantibodies (Morgan *et al.*, 1985). There are many excellent publications dealing with this matter that cannot be listed in detail, but the monograph by Campbell (1984) and the books edited by Mishell & Shiigi (1980), Springer (1985) and Weir *et al.* (1986) contain much useful general information and details of more sophisticated approaches to making MAbs. Our general procedures with an approximate timetable of events may be summarized thus:

1 Select, and purify if necessary, a suitable antigen (this is a fairly unpredictable step and is not really the subject of this chapter).
2 Immunize mice in an effective way (once relevant parameters are worked out allow 1 month).
3 Prepare lymphocyte cell suspension and mix with plasmacytoma cells in the presence of a fusogen (the day of the fusion).
4 Select the hybrids in appropriate tissue culture conditions (starting at the day of the fusion).
5 Identify monoclonal antibody-secreting cells (2 weeks after fusion).
6 Clone and grow cells as monoclonal lines (a minimum of 2 months with a repeated cycle of cloning).
7 Purify the antibody and characterize its specificity.

Thus the minimum time in which a useable reagent can be derived using our system is 3–4 months, though there are several short cuts to this recommended procedure. For instance if cloning is accomplished by limiting dilution at the fusion step, then the overall time required can be reduced considerably.

Selection, and Purification if Necessary, of a Suitable Antigen

The selection of antigen is implicit in the decision to go ahead and produce MAbs. Any decision to utilize this technology must have involved the identification of a target antigen. The techniques of cell fusion and cell cloning make possible the production of specific antibodies when the only available immunogen is impure antigen. Nevertheless, as a general rule, the purer the antigen the greater will be the proportion of derived hybridomas which secrete antibodies reactive with the required target. It must be recognized that the chance of producing MAbs against contaminants may depend upon the purity of the antigen used in the antibody screening assay (described later). Contaminants below the level of chemical detection can be powerful immunogens, and antibodies directed against them may be picked up in the screening procedure if care is not taken to exclude them. Thus the effort of purifying antigens extensively, assuming a procedure for doing so is available, may be worthwhile, although this should be balanced against the efficiency of cell cloning itself as a purification method to produce individual MAbs. For many antigens it may already be obvious how mice can be immunized optimally to produce specific serum antibody, but there are unfortunately very few general rules applicable to immunization. Thus, to produce specific MAbs the best procedure for each antigen needs to be established individually. Of course for some antigens it may not be necessary to immunize at all: in our own work we have derived many autoantibodies from animals that were never intentionally immunized. In general though, normal unimmunized mice will give rise to hybrids producing IgM of low affinity.

Immunization of Mice in an Effective Way

The purpose of any immunization schedule is to increase selectively the frequency of those lymphocytes making antibodies of the required specificity. For any given antigen there are a number of different tactics that may be used to increase the probability of producing relevant hybridomas.

Selection of mouse strain for immunization

It may be important to use animals of an inbred strain and such mice vary in their responsiveness to specific antigens. It is therefore worthwhile to screen several for their response to the antigen in question and to select the one which responds best. F_1 mice derived from different strains often respond better immunologically than homozygous parental animals. The myeloma cells commonly used to prepare hybridomas are derived from BALB/C mice. Thus, unless at least one parent of the mouse used as an immune lymphocyte donor is of BALB/C origin, particular and possibly complex histocompatibility requirements will have to be satisfied if the resultant hybridomas are to be grown as tumours in mice. Accordingly, the simplest fusion is with the immunocytes of a BALB/C mouse, so that all the hybrids will have the potential to grow within this parental strain.

Immunization schedules

It is reasonable to immunize in a way which produces a high titre of serum antibody. The resulting antiserum is of great use as a positive control in setting up a screening system for the identification of relevant MAbs. For most soluble, particulate or cellular antigens in mice this means repeated injections 1–2 weeks apart. The last injection should be given 3–4 days before cell fusion. It appears that the cell most likely to form an antibody-secreting hybrid is a preplasma cell (plasmablast) in which the antibody synthesizing machinery is activated but which has not yet undergone the irreversible cellular changes that lead to the loss of function in mature plasma cells. The last injection is given intravenously in order to deliver the antigen to the spleen. Circulating antibody levels provide only a guide to the number and specificity of antibody forming cells in the spleen. Apart from the obvious reason that the relevant cells may not be residents of the spleen there are limitations in titration systems which restrict the isotype, specificity or affinity of the antibodies detectable. Ultimately mice will need to be chosen for fusion and the most accessible of the criteria for their selection is their serum antibody status.

Immunological adjuvants and antigen modification

It may be necessary to use adjuvants to increase the number of responding lymphocytes. Oil and water emulsions allow antigen to be slowly released from a depot. Freund's Incomplete Adjuvant (FIA) is commonly used for this purpose, its adjuvant activity can be enhanced by other non-specific immunostimulatory substances such as heat-killed mycobacteria which are mixed with FIA to form Freund's Complete Adjuvant (FCA). In general, FCA is used for the first injection and FIA for the second and subsequent injections, given subcutaneously or intradermally at several different sites. Killed *Bordetella pertussis* organisms also have a strong adjuvant effect for some antigens in mice and alum-precipitated antigen may also have increased immunogenicity. It must be remembered that some adjuvants are themselves immunogenic and that they all may induce a range of antibodies that is different from that induced by antigen alone. Soluble antigens with low intrinsic immunogenicity may be linked chemically to a carrier molecule. The carrier chosen should be a T-cell dependent antigen to which the mouse itself responds well (such as bovine serum albumin).

Screening procedures

At this point it is necessary to discuss the screening procedures for the identification of MAbs secreting hybrids. The importance of this cannot be overestimated as once production is underway there will be no time available for any serious modification of an existing protocol. Individual culture wells must be tested for their ability to secrete the antibody of choice and this may involve several thousand determinations. Important considerations in the choice of assay include availability and cost of reagents, its ease and speed. We find this testing is most easily done using an enzyme linked immunosorbent assay (ELISA) system, based on the procedure originally described by Engvall & Perlmann (1972), although many other methods are available. These include radioimmunoassay, haemagglutination, complement fixation, fluorescence and precipitation in gels (though this latter option is unlikely to detect many MAbs since most do not precipitate their target antigen). There is no standard procedure and the best conditions must be empirically determined for each assay system. The most important prerequisite is a known positive control. Serum obtained by test bleeds from immunized animals, as mentioned above, can serve this function, but it is better, if possible, to use an antibody of similar reactivity to the one being sought. The assay method used will depend upon the antibody-antigen system under consideration and upon the scale of the operation. The efficiency of the screening procedure is central to the preparation of MAbs and can be the limiting factor in its success. As stated, therefore, the assay should ideally be simple, cheap, quick to perform and be able to handle large numbers of culture supernatant samples and to identify MAbs of the appropriate specificity, affinity and class. Essentially the assay should be appropriate to the use to which the MAbs ultimately will be put. Here we have chosen to describe the ELISA because if fulfils all the given requirements, and is a system which has served us well for the derivation of autoantibodies with many different specificities.

Although there is no standard ELISA system, the basic ELISA principle for the detection of specific antibody is very simple and illustrated in Fig. 1. It involves the adsorption of antigen onto a solid phase, usually a 96 well polystyrene microtitre tray; blocking the plastic against 'non-specific' binding; washing and adding the antibody to be tested; incubating, further washing and detection of specific antibody with the appropriate enzyme labelled anti-immunoglobulin reagent.

A Standard ELISA Protocol for Detection of Antibodies to a Protein Antigen

1 Prepare protein at a concentration of 10 µg/ml in sensitizing buffer (0.1 M carbonate/bicarbonate pH 9.8). Dispense 50 µl of this solution into each well of a

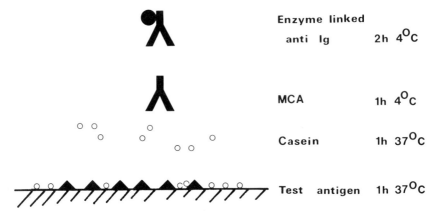

Fig. 1.   Schematic representation of a simple ELISA system used for detection of specific monoclonal antibody. (Times and temperatures at each stage are indicated.)

microtitre plate (flat bottomed rigid polystyrene Immunoplate II Nunc, Gibco U.K.). Include wells containing sensitizing buffer alone as a negative control for the protein antigen. Incubate for 1 h at 37 °C.

2 Wash the plate twice with phosphate buffered saline (PBS) pH 7.2, 0.15 M (NaCl 8.0 g/l; KCl 0.20 g/l; Na_2HPO_4 1.15 g/l; KH_2PO_4 0.20 g/l). To each well add 50 µl PBS containing 2% casein (light, white, soluble (BDH)) as blocking agent and incubate at 37 °C for 1 h.

3 Wash twice with PBS containing 0.1% Tween 20 (Sigma) (PBS-Tween). Add 50 µl of PBS containing 0.05% Tween 20 and 1% casein (PBS-C-Tween) to each well of all rows used. Add 50 µl of primary antibody to the first well of each row, mix and transfer 50 µl to next well of row, repeat along each row but discard 50 µl from the last well. Include diluent and dilutions of normal serum as negative controls. Incubate for 2 h at 4 °C.

4 Wash three times with PBS-Tween, then add to each well 50 µl of appropriate peroxidase-labelled anti-immunoglobulin reagent (Miles) diluted in PBS-C-Tween. Incubate at 4 °C for 1 h.

5 Wash plate six times with PBS-Tween. Then add to each well 50 µl of substrate/ indicator OPD (1 mg/ml ortho-phenylenediamine (BDH) dissolved in a few drops of methanol and diluted with 0.01 M citrate phosphate buffer pH 6.3: immediately before use add 1 µl/ml of 100 vols H_2O_2). Incubate for 20 min in the dark at room temperature.

6 Stop the reaction by adding 100 µl/well of 0.5 M citric acid and measure the extinction at 450 nm, then plot extinction against primary antibody dilution.

Note: with single point assays used for screening culture supernatants, the dilution step, in 3 above, is not applicable.

By calculating titre values (reciprocal antibody dilution at 50% of the maximum extinction) it is easy to compare the quality of different antibody-containing preparations. A given positive serum can be used in a chequerboard type assay to determine both the optimum antigen sensitization concentration and the optimum labelled antiglobulin concentration (see Figs. 2 and 3).

Preparation of Lymphocyte Cell Suspension and Mixture with Plasmacytoma Cells in the Presence of a Fusogen

Choice of fusion partner

Several important criteria are required to be satisfied for a myeloma to be a good fusion partner. First, such myeloma cells must inhibit neither the expression of Ig genes nor the secretion of Ig molecules in the daughter hybrid cells. Secondly, myeloma cells should not themselves secrete Ig chains but should still permit the expression of Ig genes in the complemented genome of hybrid cells derived from them. Thirdly, the myeloma cells should be sensitive to selective tissue culture conditions. Several such lines have been derived and are now commercially available. It is worth noting that the P3/NS1/1-Ag4-1 murine line (Kohler & Milstein, 1976) which is widely used does not itself secrete myeloma Ig chains but does contain intracellular κ-chains. Hybrid cells derived from it may secrete these myeloma κ-chains incorporated at random into the MAbs molecules.

Myeloma to spleen cell ratio for cell fusion

For the optimum production of hybrid cells we recommend mixing an equal number of myeloma cells with viable spleen cells. Fusion experiments were carried out in our laboratory using spleen cells from autoimmune $(NZB \times NZW)F_1$ and MRL/Mp-*1pr/1pr* strains of mice with the intention of deriving DNA-reactive MAbs. Myeloma and spleen cells were mixed at ratios of $1:1$ to $1:5$ before fusing with polyethylene glycol (PEG) and the number of cultures containing DNA-binding autoantibodies was determined. In all cases, more positive cultures were found when equal numbers of myeloma and spleen cells were used.

Fusion of Myeloma Cells (NS-1) to Mouse Spleen Cells

1 The myeloma fusion partner, P3/NS1/1-Ag4-1 (NS-1), (Flow Laboratories, Irvine, Scotland; 05-530), should be grown in RPMI 1640 medium, containing 100 units/ml penicillin, 100 μg/ml streptomycin, 2 mM glutamine and 20% fetal calf serum (RP20 medium) at 3 to 8×10^5 cells/ml. Keep the cells in the exponential phase of growth at all times leading up to the fusion event.

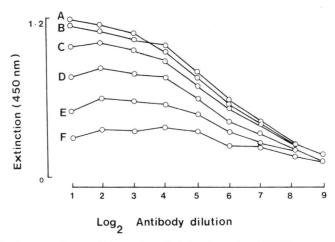

FIG. 2.   Titration curves for an anti-fibronectin antibody in a chequerboard ELISA system, as described. Each curve represents a doubling dilution of enzyme conjugated rabbit anti-mouse IgG, where the most concentrated, A, is a 1/100 dilution of the original reagent. It is clear that dilution greater than 1/400 (curve C), gives suboptimal activity.

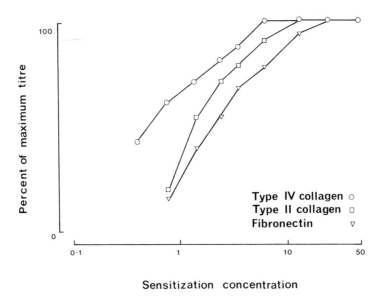

FIG. 3.   A chequerboard ELISA between the concentration of sensitizing antigen and the primary antibody for three different antigens. Antibody titres (see text) at each sensitization concentration were plotted as a percentage of the maximum titre so that the optimum sensitization concentration for each antigen is clearly revealed.

2 Prepare a 50% solution of polyethylene glycol (PEG) molecular weight 1500 (AnalaR, BDH, Dorset): autoclave for 20 min at 15 psi, then add 1 ml warm RPMI 1640 medium containing 100 units/ml penicillin, 100 μg/ml streptomycin, 2 mM glutamine (RP medium) to 1 g sterile PEG solution.

3 Immediately prior to fusion, count the NS-1 cells using white cell counting fluid (0.1 M acetic acid with enough Crystal Violet to colour the solution) and assess their viability using Trypan Blue (0.2% Trypan Blue in saline (Sigma), filter before use) dye exclusion (it should be $> 95\%$). Wash three times, by centrifugation 500 g/ 10 min/room temperature, in RP medium to remove the serum.

4 Kill the mice by cervical dislocation, submerge them in 70% alcohol and place them in a sterile area to dry. Remove the spleen and prepare a cell suspension as quickly as possible in RP medium. Count the immune spleen cell suspension for fusion and assess its viability. Mix the immune spleen cells with the NS-1 cells at a ratio of 1:1. Centrifuge 500 g for 10 min at room temperature and remove the supernatant. Normal feeder cells will also be required so prepare a normal spleen cell suspension in RP20 medium and keep it aside at 37 °C. Use one feeder spleen with every experimental spleen.

5 Add 1 ml PEG 50%, at 37 °C, to the drained cell pellet over 60 s mixing well. Incubate the cells at 37 °C for 60 s and then slowly dilute with RP medium, adding the first 1 ml over 60 s and a further 9 ml over 5 min. Centrifuge the mixture, 500 g for 5 min at room temperature and resuspend the pellet in RP20 containing HAT supplement (1×10^{-4} M hypoxanthine, 1.6×10^{-5} M thymidine and 4×10^{-7} M aminopterin) and the feeder spleen cells. Plate out into 24 well plates, (Gibco) at 1– 10×10^5 (depending on experiment) original spleen cells per well and transfer to 37 °C 5% CO_2 incubator until growth is visible.

6 The cultures should show macroscopic growth after 7 to 11 days and can then be screened for antibody production. They should be fed at this stage with RP20 medium containing HAT supplement. This is accomplished by removing half the medium (most easily done with a vacuum line attached to a side arm flask) and replacing it with fresh medium. The cultures should then be fed with RP20 whenever the medium is acid (i.e. yellow).

Selection of the Hybrids in Appropriate Tissue Culture Conditions

Positive selection of hybridized lymphocytes in culture

After the fusion event a number of viable cell combinations exist: fused myeloma X B-cells, unfused myeloma cells and a mixed group of non-functionally fused cells. The selection procedure is designed to remove all non-relevant cells so that only the correctly fused myeloma X B-cells remain. Unfused spleen cells have a relatively short life and most will die in culture during the first week. The myeloma X non-

B-cells have intrinsically low viability and are generally of no significance. The major contaminant is therefore the unfused myeloma cells. Selection against these cells is dependent upon using a cell line which lacks the enzyme hypoxanthine guanine phosphoribosyl transferase (HGPRT⁻) which is an enzyme involved in the scavenger (or rescue) pathway of DNA synthesis. If the other pathway of DNA synthesis, the *de novo* pathway, is blocked by the folic acid reductase antagonist aminopterin, only cells able to use the scavenger pathway, i.e. the fused cells (now HGPRT⁺), can survive if they are provided with hypoxanthine and thymidine. The cells surviving the fusion and selection procedure are, therefore, likely to be functionally fused myeloma X B-cells and a high percentage will produce immunoglobulin. The overall frequency of formation of viable hybrid cells is, however, low. Most cells die at an early stage and this can be indirectly damaging to the surviving cells. Because of this the cultures are supplemented, directly after fusion and before plating out, with a normal feeder cell population and are then left undisturbed for up to 1 week after fusion. Many different cell types are commonly used as feeders, e.g. spleen cells, thymus cells, peritoneal exudate cells (PEC), erythrocytes or irradiated fibroblasts. All effectively increase the survival of hybrid cells, though the macrophages in peritoneal exudate or spleen cells have an added advantage in that they phagocytose cell debris from the cultures. We use a feeder spleen in the initial fusion procedure and thereafter peritoneal macrophages when cloning or if the cells have overgrown and died back.

Culture conditions

Hybrid lymphocytes are cultured under standard tissue culture (TC) conditions. Because of the cost and periodic scarcity of fetal calf serum (FCS) there can be advantages in using other serum sources such as horse, pig or newborn calf. In each case, the serum must be free of virus and *Mycoplasma* contamination and should be screened for toxicity against at least the parent myeloma and also, if possible, some hybridoma lines. The most sensitive measure of serum toxicity is its effect upon cell cloning efficiency although a reasonable approximation may be achieved by determining its effect upon logarithmic growth rates of cloned cells. Additionally, all TC sera should be checked for potential interference in the assay systems to be used in screening for antibody production by hybrid cells. This is particularly important with TC sera, other than FCS, which contain immunoglobulin.

The initial distribution of fused cells into many small cultures is a first step towards separating clones of hybrid cells from each other. After a few days, small clonal growth foci (cloids) are visible in the multi-well cultures and if the fused cell mixture has been diluted correctly there will be only a few clones growing in each culture. Not all clones growing in HAT medium secrete specific MAbs. Some are HGPRT⁺ revertant myeloma cells (arising at a rate of 10^{-5} to 10^{-6}) but most are hybrid cells, the majority of which secrete monoclonal immunoglobulins of unknown specificity rather than of the required specificity against the immunizing antigen.

The number of clones that can be derived from a single fusion depends upon many factors and varies in a complex way with cell concentration, culture volume and the feeder cell type. As a guide, 10^8 spleen lymphocytes fused with 10^8 NS-1 myeloma cells and plated (with an equivalent number of normal spleen feeder cells) into 480 2 ml cultures may produce up to 50 cloids per culture within 2 weeks. It is, of course, impossible to give a meaningful estimate of the number of clones likely to be secreting antibodies of a given specificity. This will vary according to the immune state of the animal and the fusion efficiency.

Hybridoma cells are not tolerant of alkaline culture conditions and should therefore be maintained in an atmosphere containing at least 5% CO_2. Culture media, resupplemented with fresh glutamine, should be used to feed the growing cells each week or whenever the medium is acid.

Identification of Monoclonal Antibody Secreting Cells

Individual culture wells must be tested for their ability to secrete the antibody of choice, as described above (p. 5).

Cloning and Growing Cells as Monoclonal Lines

Having screened the cultures for antibody production, it is then necessary to separate a stable clone of cells producing the required antibody from the many other hybrid cells that will also be growing in it. One way this cloning can be achieved is by growing the cells at limiting dilution using peritoneal exudate cells (PEC) as a feeder layer. The cell cultures can then be expanded and implanted into pristane primed syngeneic mice to produce ascitic fluid. We have found that cloning by limiting dilution using PEC as feeder cells is the most efficient and successful method (Fig. 4).

Collection of feeder cells

1 Inject 0.5 ml pristane (2, 6, 10, 14 tetra methyl pentadecane, Aldrich) intraperitoneally into mice allowing one mouse per ten 96 well TC microtitre plates.
2 Three weeks later anaesthetize each mouse with ether and swab the abdomen with 70% alcohol. Allow the alcohol to evaporate off under a lamp, while maintaining anaesthesia.
3 Inject 5 ml of culture medium (RP20) intraperitoneally, massage the abdomen and remove the medium with a syringe and a new 21 gauge needle.

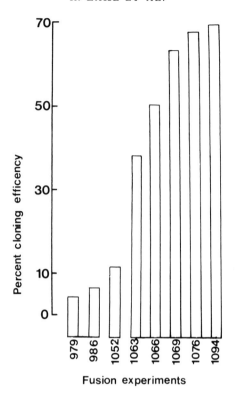

Fig. 4.   Cloning efficiency in eight sequential fusion experiments. Cloning efficiency is calculated as the number of established stable cell lines expressed as a percentage of the number of cultures found initially in that fusion experiment. Eight fusion experiments were carried out using spleen cells from autoimmune mice. Cultures containing cells that produced DNA-binding autoantibodies from fusions 979 and 986 were cloned using semi-solid agarose and less than 10% became stable cell lines. Cells from fusion 1052 were cloned by limiting dilution but without feeder cells and 12% became stable cell lines. The cloning efficiency improved from 40% to 70% using our recommended procedure (see text) from fusion 1063 to 1094.

Cloning method

Cells can be cloned at limit dilution either with the feeder cells mixed in with the diluent or onto plates already seeded with these cells. The relative advantages of the two techniques are the speed of the former, where only a single plating out operation is required, versus the ability to identify contaminated feeders in the latter case, which is described here.

1 Plate out the feeder cells in 100 μl volumes of RP20 into each well of a 96 well TC plate so as to get about 10^4 feeder cells per well. The plates can then be left at 37 °C for up to 1 week.

2 Mix the suspension of cells to be cloned and prepare 30 ml of culture medium containing 30 cells/ml. Ensure the suspension is thoroughly mixed, avoiding air bubbles.

3 Take 20 ml of this suspension and (with a multichannel pipette) distribute 100 µl/well into two of the 96 well TC plates.

4 Dilute the remaining cells to 10 cells/ml and repeat.

5 Dilute the remainder to 3 cells/ml and plate them out similarly.

6 Incubate the cells with minimal disturbance at 37 °C, in an atmosphere of 5% CO_2 in air for 10–14 days or until visible clones appear.

7 Feed the cells by adding 100 µl of fresh medium to each well and reincubate. Assay, feed and/or reclone as required.

8 Calculate the percent of negative wells (for both growth and antibody production) at each of the cell concentrations originally plated out.

A semi-logarithmic plot of the percentage of negative wells against the original cell number plated out is a convenient way of estimating the likelihood of monclonality and the clonal characteristics of a particular cell line. The number of cells originally plated out that gives rise to an average of one cell per well (either growing or secreting antibody) is given by the interpolated value at the level of 37% negative cultures, this value comes from the Poisson formula (limiting dilution analysis is well discussed by Lefkovits & Waldmann, 1979). Figure 5 shows limiting dilution analyses for several DNA-reactive MAbs. Some lines will never be truly monoclonal, in the sense that a certain percentage of cells at each generation lose the ability to either synthesize or secrete MAbs. Such lines need to be more carefully handled and regularly recloned. Probably the most important criterion for judging monoclonality rests with the distinction between the two lines drawn from the data regarding growth and that regarding antibody production. Essentially a cell line can only be regarded as monoclonal if all cultures at limiting dilution secrete antibody.

Purification of the Antibody and Characterization of its Specificity

Growing hybrid cell lines and harvesting MAbs

By the very process of their selection, hybridomas are usually well adapted to grow *in vitro*. If conventional TC media supplemented with sera are used, the spent medium will contain typically 1–10 µg/ml specific MAbs if the hybridoma cells have been allowed to grow to exhaustion. When MAbs derived in this way are used for experiment or assay, the presence of large amounts of heterologous serum protein in the spent TC media may be undesirable for both technical and economic reasons. Hybridomas can be adapted to grow in low concentrations of serum, sometimes less than 1%, by gradually reducing the serum concentration over several days or weeks of culture. In general, lower serum concentrations cause a

Cell number per well

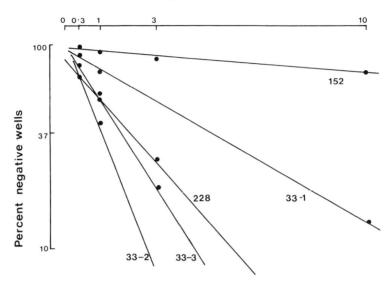

FIG. 5.   Limiting dilution analyses of several different cell lines secreting DNA-reactive antibodies. The percentage of wells not producing antibody is plotted against the original number of cells plated out in each well. Line I-33 was sequentially cloned (33-2) 6 weeks after initial cloning (33-1) and again (33-3) 10 weeks later. It is clear that the number of cells required for an average one antibody forming unit per well varies, so that only the second cloning of line 33 (33-2) shows good evidence of monoclonality, the trivial explanation for a greater than one cell per well requirement is a poor initial viability.

reduced growth rate and support a lower maximum cell density, though not necessarily affecting the amount of antibody elaborated into the medium. Most cloned hybrid lymphocytes will grow as tumours in appropriate animals—a property they share with the parent myeloma lines—hence the derivation of the term *hybridoma*. Cells are implanted subcutaneously or intraperitoneally. The dose of cells required for a successful 'take', often initially in excess of 10^7, will decrease if the cell line becomes adapted for *in vivo* growth by repeated passage. Such lines must be checked frequently for antibody secretion whether they are maintained either by *in vivo* passage or by *in vitro* culture. Hybridoma cells form a palpable tumour within 2 weeks of subcutaneous implantation and antibody accumulates in the blood. Hybridomas isolated early after fusion often grow better subcutaneously than intraperitoneally. However, most lines when implanted in the latter site induce accumulation of ascites fluid containing MAbs (at up to 10 mg/ml) which will also be present at a similar level in the serum. Ascites fluid accumulation and intraperitoneal tumour growth can be enhanced by priming mice with light mineral oil (intraperitoneal injection of 0.5 ml, 3 weeks before cells, see method for induction of PEC, p. 11). Cells are implanted intraperitoneally when oil-induced fluid starts to accumulate in the peritoneal cavity. Monoclonal antibodies may reach concentrations of 10 mg/ml in ascites fluid and repeated drainage of the peritoneal cavity can provide more than 10 ml of fluid from each mouse. The obvious advantage of growing a hybridoma *in vivo* is the amount of antibody produced, but this will be contaminated with normal mouse immunoglobulin which may not be acceptable in all situations.

Purification of MAbs

For many applications MAbs need not be recovered from culture media or ascites fluids. If purification is required then several procedures are available for this. Monoclonal antibodies can be purified from ascites fluids or culture supernatant by affinity chromatography using either specific antigen linked to Sepharose or more generally protein A Sepharose (Pharmacia).

Purification from ascites fluid

1 Collect ascites fluid and allow it to clot. Separate the serum by centrifugation (1000 g for 10 min at room temperature) and store it in aliquots at -20 °C.
2 Dilute 2 ml of this fluid with an equal volume of phosphate buffer (0.1 M, pH 8.0) and pass it through a column containing Sepharose 4B (a 5 ml syringe barrel makes a convenient column). This will remove any proteins that bind directly to Sepharose and ensure that the solution is free of aggregate which could contaminate the more valuable affinity column.
3 Pass this filtered material through a similar protein A Sepharose (Sigma) column several times. Wash out any material not adsorbed onto the protein A Sepharose with at least 30 ml of phosphate buffer (0.1 M, pH 8.0).
4 Elute the adsorbed antibody with citrate-phosphate buffer (0.1 M, pH 2.8 and pH 6.0 for IgG_2 and IgG_1 antibodies respectively), this is easily accomplished by gently layering the new buffer onto the drained gel bed surface. Monitor the eluate spectrophotometrically and neutralize it immediately with saturated Tris solution.
5 Dialyse the affinity purified material into phosphate buffered saline (PBS) by gel-filtration using a Sephadex G25 column (Pharmacia).
6 Store aliquots of purified antibodies at -20 °C.

Purification of MAbs from culture supernatants

1 Concentrate supernatants from cultures containing cells secreting monoclonal antibodies by salt precipitation. Slowly add solid ammonium sulphate to culture supernatant while stirring until 45% saturation is achieved.
2 Separate the resulting precipitate by centrifugation 2000 g for 15 min at room temperature and then rewash with 45% saturated ammonium sulphate. Resuspend

the washed precipitate in a minimum of 0.8% saline and dialyse it into phosphate buffer (0.1 M, pH 8.0).

The precipitable material from culture supernatants will contain a mixture of proteins including monoclonal antibody from the cell line and bovine immunoglobulin from the calf serum. Monoclonal antibodies from culture supernatants can be purified from this material by affinity chromatography using protein A Sepharose in the same way as the ascitic fluids. For some uses it may be necessary to remove bovine immunoglobulin using an anti-bovine immunoglobulin immunoadsorbent column.

Isotype determination

A required isotype may be central to the success of a particular strategy and, in addition, isotype determination is essential to the design of appropriate purification procedures. The biological activities of different heavy chains (isotype determining regions) are well described in most immunology texts and these activities will be relevant even if the antibody is to be used solely *in vitro*. For example, many assay systems depend upon complement consumption and different classes of antibody do not fix complement equally. In general, IgM antibodies are less desirable because of their instability, low intrinsic affinity and the problems associated with purifying them.

The isotype of MAbs can be readily determined with an adaptation of the ELISA system already described. A three-stage system is used. Wells are sensitized with antigen and blocked. The lowest concentration of antibody that gives maximum binding, previously established, is added followed by dilutions of rabbit anti-isotype reagent (Miles). The assay is completed with the relevant conjugated antiglobulin. The isotype of five DNA-binding autoantibodies was determined using this method (Fig. 6). Four were found to be IgG_{2a} and one IgG_{2b}.

Specificity of MAbs

The apparent specificity of antibodies can change with the physicochemical properties of assay systems. Thus, the functional specificity of each MAbs must be determined for each assay system used. For example one DNA-binding autoantibody (I-33) binds to DNA when it is immobilized on a solid-phase (ELISA) but will not precipitate labelled DNA from a fluid-phase (Farr type) assay. The antigen specificity of MAbs can be determined in two ways. The comparative direct binding titres of MAbs to different antigens may reflect the relative preference of one MAb for a particular antigen. However, the direct titre in ELISA will be affected by the concentration of antigen on the plastic, in turn a function of its ability to stick to plastic and the density of epitopes on the molecule. It may be more appropriate to

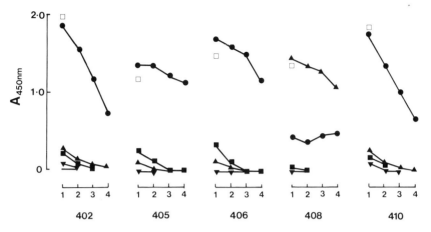

Fig. 6. Isotype of five DNA-binding autoantibodies. A constant amount of each MAb was bound to DNA in an ELISA. Dilutions of rabbit anti-isotype specific reagents (1, 1/250; 2, 1/500; 3, 1/1000; 4, 1/2000) were added and the assay completed as described (see text). Absorbance at 450 nm is plotted against dilutions of anti-isotype antibodies: (■), anti-IgG$_1$; (●), anti-IgG$_{2a}$; (▲), anti-IgG$_{2b}$; (□), anti-IgG$_{H+L}$. Anti-IgG$_3$ and anti-IgM reagents were used but antibodies of these isotypes were not found.

measure the inhibitory potency of antigens by their ability to compete for the MAbs. The concentration of antibody that gives 60–70% maximum binding is established in a direct ELISA as described above. Serial dilutions of inhibitors are then used to inhibit this binding. Results are expressed as the concentration of inhibitor required for 50% inhibition of the binding of the antibodies. Three MAbs that bind to DNA in the DNA-binding ELISA were found to have distinct ligand binding properties using an inhibition system (Fig. 7). Monoclonal antibody I-33 bound preferentially to dsDNA, MAb IV-228 exclusively to ssDNA and MAb V-88 to ssDNA, dsDNA and RNA in decreasing order of preference. The examples quoted here are taken from Morgan *et al.* (1985).

Labelling MAbs

Many protocols exist for external labelling of both serum and monoclonal antibodies with a fluorochrome, an enzyme (e.g. horseradish peroxidase or alkaline phosphatase) or with a radionuclide. The success of any one particular method of external labelling cannot be guaranteed, though MAbs have one considerable advantage over conventional serum antibodies in that they can be easily labelled internally with one or a number of [3]H- or ^{14}C-labelled amino acids by growing the hybridoma cells for up to 24 h in an appropriate TC medium containing such labelled precursors. These antibodies are particularly useful for immunochemical and immunocyto-chemical procedures and have the advantage of retaining their native conformation.

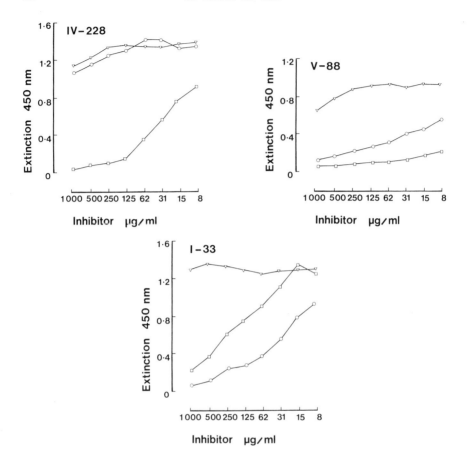

Fɪɢ. 7. Specificity of DNA-binding autoantibodies. The ligand binding properties of three DNA-binding autoantibodies were determined using an inhibition ELISA system. Free (○) dsDNA; (□) ssDNA; and (▽) RNA were used to inhibit the binding to bound ssDNA, for autoantibodies IV-228 and V-88, and to bound dsDNA in the case of I-33.

Internal labelling of MAbs

1 Grow hybridoma cells exponentially under standard TC conditions.
2 Wash an aliquot of 10^6 cells in RPMI without phenylalanine (RP⁻) medium (RPMI Selectamine Gibco) by centrifugation 500 g for 10 min at room temperature.
3 Resuspend the cells in 1 ml of RP⁻ medium supplemented with 10 μCi of ^{14}C labelled phenylalanine (Amersham).
4 Return the culture to a humidified 5% CO_2 atmosphere at 37 °C for 18 h.
5 Centrifuge 1000 g for 10 min at room temperature. Remove the supernatant, purify the antibody if required and store it at − 20 °C.

References

CAMPBELL, A. 1984 Monoclonal antibody technology. *Laboratory Techniques in Biochemistry & Molecular Biology* Vol. 13. London: Elsevier.

ENGVALL, E. & PERLMANN, P. 1972 Enzyme linked immunosorbent assay ELISA III. Quantitation of specific antibodies by enzyme labelled anti-immunoglobulin in antigen coated tubes. *Journal of Immunology* 109, 129–135.

KOHLER, G. & MILSTEIN, C. 1976 Derivation of specific antibody-producing tissue culture and tumour lines by cell fusion. *European Journal of Immunology* 6, 511–519.

LEFKOVITS, I. & WALDMANN, H. 1979 *Limiting Dilution Analysis of Cells in the Immune System*. Cambridge: Cambridge University Press.

MISHELL, B. & SHIIGI, S. (Eds) 1980 *Selected Methods in Cellular Immunology*. San Francisco: W. H. Freeman & Co.

MORGAN, A., BUCHANNAN, R., LEW, A., OLSEN, I. & STAINES, N. 1985 Five groups of antigenic determinants on DNA identified by monoclonal antibodies from (NZB × NZW)F₁ and MRL/Mp-1*pr*/1*pr* mice. *Immunology* 55, 75–83.

SPRINGER, T. (Ed) 1985 *Hybridoma Technology in the Biosciences and Medicine*. New York: Plenum Press.

WEIR, D., BLACKWELL, C., HERZENBERG, L. & HERZENBERG, L. (Eds) 1986 *Handbook of Experimental Immunology*. Oxford: Blackwell Scientific Publications.

Purification and Analysis of Monoclonal Antibodies from Mouse Ascites Fluid by High Performance Ion-Exchange and Size-Exclusion Chromatography

JOHN H. CREEDY

LKB Instruments Ltd, 232 Addington Road, Selsdon, Surrey CR2 8YD

Introduction

Monoclonal antibodies are currently of great interest for use both as *in vitro* and *in vivo* diagnostic and therapeutic agents. Many chromatographic purification procedures have been suggested and successfully applied, such as anion exchange (Burchiel *et al.*, 1984), protein A gel (Goding, 1978), hydroxyapatite (Stanker *et al.*, 1985), hydrophobic interaction (Pavlu *et al.*, 1985), DEAE affigel blue (Bruck *et al.*, 1982) and cation exchange (Carlsson *et al.*, 1985). None of these methods can truly be applied generally, however, because of the heterogeneity in the isoelectric point, hydrophobicity and size as well as in the biological activity of different monoclonal antibodies. Furthermore, the nature of the medium, in which the monoclonal antibody is present, is of importance.

The choice of method(s) must therefore be optimized for the monoclonal antibody to be purified and also for the amount of material purified at each time. The HPLC methodology is well suited for up to gram amounts while large scale methods are used when kilograms of material have to be processed.

Our aim with this study was to improve the purification of monoclonal antibodies from mouse ascites fluids. (These antibodies are used for diagnostic tests that LKB are currently manufacturing.) Our objectives were to:

1 improve purity,
2 simplify the method,
3 increase reproducibility,
4 suggest automation possibilities for producing more than 100 mg of pure antibody at each time.

Material and Methods

Production of monoclonal antibodies (MAbs)

The MAbs (IgG_1 and IgM) were prepared by the LKB microbiology group essentially according to the technique described by de St. Groth *et al.* (1980).

Immunological Techniques
in Microbiology

Treatment of ascites fluid

The ascites fluids were centrifuged at $1940 \times g$ for 15 min and then the supernatants were passed through 0.2 μm filters (Millipore). This procedure was necessary in order to maintain the lifetime of the columns.

Chromatographic procedure

The chromatographic conditions are described in each figure except the comparison with a protein A gel purification shown in Fig. 1B, 1C. The protein A purification was performed on a Protein A-Ultrogel column (25 ml) (LKB-Produkter AB). The starting buffer was 10 mM phosphate buffer, pH 8.6, at a flow rate of 0.4 ml/min, and the eluent buffer consisted of 10 mM citric acid, pH 2.5, containing 0.5 M NaCl.

Activity and purity analysis

The activity of the MAbs was determined by enzyme-linked immunosorbent assay (ELISA) in all peak fractions (Absorbtion 280 nm). The microtitration plates that were used consist of 96 flat bottomed wells for spectrophotometric reading on ELISA meters.

The total protein contents of the collected fractions were determined according to Bradford (1976) with reagents from Bio-Rad Laboratories, München, West Germany.

Polyacrylamide gel electrophoresis (PAGE) was performed under reducing conditions in sodium dodecyl sulphate (SDS) according to the method of Laemmli (1970). A 4% stacking gel was used to load samples on a 12% separating gel. Gels were stained with Coomassie Brilliant Blue R250 (LKB-Produkter AB).

The peak fractions from the cation exchange separations of the MAbs of IgG_1 type have also been analysed by isoelectric focussing. The focussing was performed in an agarose gel (0.5 mm). Only the immunoglobulins were stained by an immunofixation procedure in the main according to Santana (1983).

Choice of instrumentation

The hardware associated with this general type of biologically active preparative purification demands special consideration. It is well documented that stainless steel corrodes significantly in the presence of buffer systems, notably those containing halide ions. This introduces both ferric ions and heavy metals such as chromium into solution. In the case of a chromatography fluidic system the yield from this precolumn corrosion all inevitably passes through the column where chelation may occur. Samples that subsequently pass through such a column are thus exposed to unusually and progressively high levels of such contaminants. Many biologically active molecules are adversely affected to a greater or lesser extent by such exposure. The recommendation, thus, is to avoid any unnecessary contact with sources of such contamination wherever possible. For this reason, and also for the reason that the hardware itself can be rendered unreliable and, at worst, inoperable by such corrosion, it was decided to employ glass packed columns with teflon frits, titanium or teflon tubing and connectors and, most significantly, an HPLC pump and detector flow cell constructed entirely of titanium at all metal/fluid interfaces.

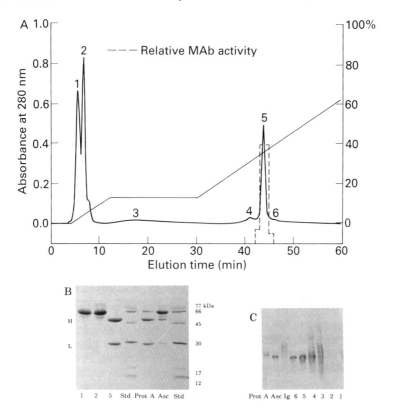

Fig. 1.   Purification of IgG$_1$ monoclonal antibodies. (A) Purification of mouse IgG$_1$ monoclonal antibody present in ascites fluid on a cation exchange column. (B) Eluted peaks were treated with SDS and subjected to electrophoresis under reducing conditions on a 12% SDS-polyacrylamide gel. Numbers below each lane correspond to peak numbers. Std = molecular weight standards; Asc = ascites fluid with the IgG$_1$ 1 MAbs; Prot A = protein A purified MAbs (IgG$_1$) H = heavy chains; L = light chains. (C) Eluted peaks were also analysed with isoelectric focusing/immunofixation. Numbers below each lane correspond to peak numbers. Ig = mouse IgG; Asc = ascites fluid with the (IgG$_1$) MAbs; Prot A = protein A purified MAbs (IgG$_1$). **Conditions:** Sample: 200 μl ascites (4 mg protein). Buffer A: 10 mM phosphate buffer adj to pH 6.4. Buffer B: 1.0 M NaCl in 10 mM phosphate buffer adj to pH 6.4. Flow rate: 0.5 ml/min. Columns: LKB 2133-065 GlasPac TSK SP-5PW. Guard Kit. LKB 2133-510 GlasPac TSK SP-5PW. (Further details are available from the author.)

Results and Discussion

Purification of IgG₁ monoclonal antibodies

A monoclonal antibody of IgG_1 class for diagnostic use was purified on a cation exchange column. This chromatographic method was chosen because of the isoelectric point of the MAb (approximately 7.5) which makes it possible to bind it at pH 6.4 while the main part of the impurities is eluted with the void volume: 200 μl pure ascites fluid was analysed and gave the chromatogram shown in Fig. 1A. The purity was checked with SDS-PAGE (Fig. 1B) and isoelectric focussing (Fig. 1C). The late-eluting peak contained the desired MAb with no detectable impurities (such as albumin, transferrin and host immunoglobulins). Recovery of biological activity was determined by ELISA to be 80%. In this case, it was possible to achieve a desired pure MAb with only one step.

This procedure was compared with purification on Protein A gel. The purity, checked with SDS-PAGE (Fig. 1B), indicates lower values than with cation exchange chromatography, and the recovery was only 45%.

Automatic repetitive purification of IgG₁ monoclonal antibodies

For further diagnostic studies larger quantities (> 10 mg) of MAbs are needed. To scale up there are two possible alternatives.

1 Utilize a larger column.
2 Make repetitive injections on an analytical sized column.

In this study we chose automatic repetitive injection since we did not need to change any parameter and we could use the same analytical HPLC system. A schematic drawing of the system is shown in Fig. 2; 1 ml ascites fluid, diluted 1:1 in starting buffer, was automatically injected repetitively for 25 h. The dilution in this case was made to reduce viscosity. One of the chromatograms obtained is shown in Fig. 3A.

The high reproducibility of the method (SD < 0.4% in retention time) allowed for collection of the MAbs with the aid of a level sensor into one single tube. In this case 10 mg of pure MAb was obtained and the purity was also checked with size exclusion chromatography (Fig. 3B) which is a fast and simple method.

Purification of IgM monoclonal antibodies with an automated 2-column switching technique

A MAb of the IgM class was also purified with cation exchange chromatography. In this case, however, the desired purity could not be achieved in one single chromatographic step (Fig. 4), therefore a second step had to be introduced. Size exclusion on a GlasPac column G4000SW was chosen since the size of the IgM

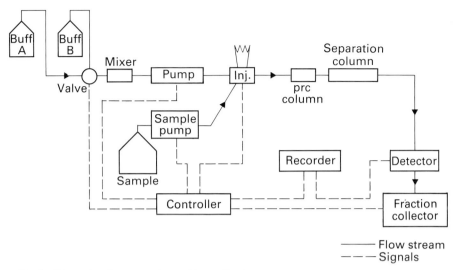

FIG. 2.   Schematics of an automatic repetitive purification system.

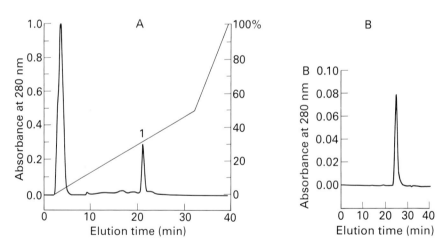

FIG. 3.   Automatic repetitive purification of IgG₁ monoclonal antibodies. (A) Automatic repetitive purification of mouse IgG₁ monoclonal antibody present in ascites fluid on a cation exchange column. **Conditions (A):** Sample: 100 μl ascites diluted 1:1 with starting buffer (14 mg protein). Buffer A: 10 mM phosphate buffer adj to pH 6.4. Buffer B: 1.0 M NaCl in 10mM phosphate buffer adj to pH 6.4. Flow rate: 1 ml/min. Columns: LKB 2133-065 GlasPac TSK SP-5PW. Guard Kit. LKB 2133-510 GlasPac TSK SP-5PW. (B) The purity of the eluted MAb (IgG₁) was checked by size exclusion. **Conditions (B):** Sample: 200 μl from peak 1 (0.11 mg protein). Eluent: 100 mM phosphate buffer adj to pH 6.4. Flow rate: 0.5 ml/min. Columns: LKB 2135-840 GlasPac TSK G4000SW.

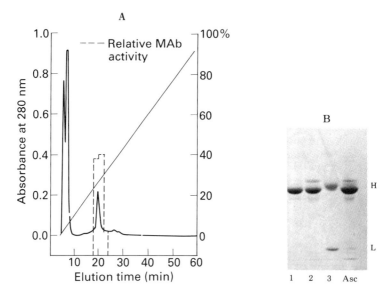

FIG. 4. Purification of IgM monoclonal antibodies. (A) Purification of mouse IgM monoclonal antibody present in ascites fluid on a cation exchange column. (B) Eluted peaks were treated with SDS and subjected to electrophoresis under reducing conditions. Numbers below each lane correspond to peak numbers. Asc = ascites fluid with the IgM MAbs; H = heavy chains; L = light chains. **Conditions:** Sample: 200 μl ascites (5 mg protein). Buffer A: 10 mM phosphate buffer adj to pH 6.4. Buffer B: 1.0 M NaCl in 10 mM phosphate buffer adj to pH 6.4. Flow rate: 0.5 ml/min. Columns: LKB 2133-065 GlasPac TSK SP-5PW. Guard Kit. LKB 2133-510 GlasPac TSK SP-5PW.

molecule (approximately 900 Kd) is bigger than most of the impurities and, to make this procedure automatic, a 2-column switching device was used.

The MAb was bound to the cation exchange column, the unbound material was discarded. A step-gradient was applied after 12 min and the switching device was connected to the size exclusion column. Figure 5 shows a schematic drawing of this system. In Fig. 6A the results after these two steps are shown. The desired purity was obtained and the biological recovery was approximately 100% in each chromatographic step. Figure 6B shows the result when no size exclusion column was used.

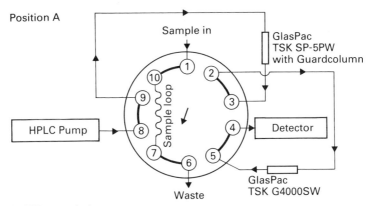

Position A: Fill sample loop

Position B: Inject sample on GlasPac TSK SP-5PW column.

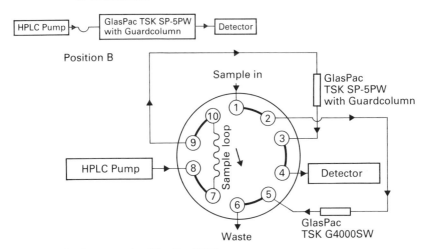

Position A: Connect the GlasPac TSK G4000SW column in series with the GlasPac TSK SP-5PW column.

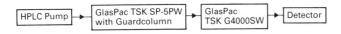

FIG. 5.   Schematics of an automated 2-column switching technique.

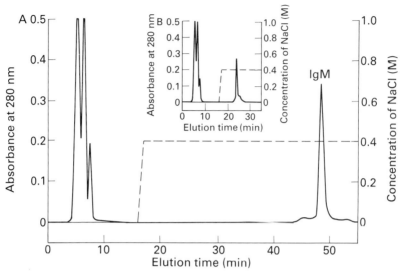

FIG. 6.   Automated 2-column switching technique for purification of IgM monoclonal antibodies. (A) Purification of mouse IgM monoclonal antibody from ascites fluid. After binding to a cation exchange column the IgM peak is eluted and transferred to a size exclusion column. (B) Purification of mouse IgM monoclonal antibody present in ascites fluid on a cation exchange column when no size exclusion column is used. **Conditions:** Sample: 100 μl ascites (2.5 mg protein). Buffer A: 10 mM phosphate buffer adj to pH 6.4. Buffer B: 1.0 M NaCl in 10 mM phosphate buffer adj to pH 6.4. Flow rate: 0.5 ml/min. Columns: LKB 2133-065 GlasPac TSK SP-5PW. Guard Kit. LKB 2133-510 GlasPac TSK SP-5PW. LKB 2135-840 GlasPac TSK G4000SW. (Further details are available from the author.)

Appendix

Instrumentation

Chromatography

Solvent delivery	LKB 2150–020 GTi Pump.
Sample application	LKB 2154–002 Injector (used in the manual gradient system).
	LKB 2154–003 10 port motorized valve (used in the repetitive and the automatic column switching system).
Gradient formation	LKB 2152–010 LC Controller.
Detector	LKB 2158–010 Uvicord SD Fixed Wavelength Detector.
Recorder	LKB 2240–020 Alphaplot Printer Plotter (2-channel).
Fraction collector	LKB 221–010 Helirac Fraction Collector.

The components below were added to configure the automatic repetitive system:

LKB 2232–002 MicroPerpex S. Peristaltic Pump.
LKB 2212–202 Level Sensor.
LKB 2220–002 Recording Integrator.

Electrophoresis

Electrophoresis unit	LKB 2001–001 Vertical Electrophoresis Unit.
Power supply	LKB 2197–022 Power Supply.
Cooling unit	LKB 2209–002 Multitemp Thermostatic Circulator.
Reagents	LKB 1820–101 UltroGrade Acrylamide.
	LKB 1830–101 Sodium Dodecyl Sulphate.
	LKB 1830–801 Tris.
	LKB 1840–101 Coomassie Bluc R 250.

Isoelectrofocussing

Electrofocussing unit	LKB 2217–001 Ultrophor Electrofocussing Unit.
Power supply	LKB 2197–022 Power Supply.
Cooling unit	LKB 2209–002 Multitemp Thermostatic Circulator.
Reagents	LKB 2206–111 Isogel Agarose-EF.
	LKB 1818–101 Ampholine EF, pH 3.5–9.5.

References

BRADFORD, M. 1976 A rapid and sensitive method for the quantitation of microgram quantities of protein using the principle of protein dyc binding. *Analytical Biochemistry* 72, 248–254.

BRUCK, C., PORTETELLE, D., GLINEUR, C. & BOLLEN, A. 1982 One step purification of mouse monoclonal antibodies from ascitic fluid by DEAE Affi-Gel Blue Chromatography. *Journal of Immunological Methods* 53, 313–319.

BURCHIEL, S. W., BILLMAN, J. R. & ALBER, T. R. 1984 Rapid and efficient purification of mouse monoclonal antibodies from ascites fluid using high performance liquid chromatography. *Journal of Immunological Methods* 69, 33–42.

CARLSSON, M., HEDIN, A., INGANAS, M., HARFAST, B. & BLOMBERG, F. 1985 Purification of *in vitro* produced mouse monoclonal antibodies. A two step procedure utilizing cation exchange chromatography. *Journal of Immunological Methods* 79, 89–98.

DE ST. GROTH, S. F. & SCHEIDEGGER, D. 1980 Production of monoclonal antibodies: strategy and tactics. *Journal of Immunological Methods* 35, 1–21.

GODING, J. W. 1978 Use of staphylococcal protein A as an immunological reagent. *Journal of Immunological Methods* 20, 241–253.

LAEMMLI, U. K. 1970 Cleavage of structural proteins during the assembly of the head of bacteriophage T4. *Nature* 227, 680–685.

PAVLU, B., JOHANSSON, U., NYHLEN, C. & WICKMAN, A. 1985 Rapid purification of monoclonal antibodies by high performance liquid chromatography. *Fifth International Symposium on HPLC of Proteins, Peptides and Polynucleotides.* Toronto, November 4–6.

SANTANA, R. 1983 Letter to the Editor. *Journal of Immunological Methods* 61, 129–130.

STANKER, L. H., VANDERLAAN, M. & JUAREZ-SALINAS, H. 1985 One step purification of mouse monoclonal antibodies from ascites fluid by hydroxyapatite chromatography. *Journal of Immunological Methods* 76, 157–169.

Measurements of Specific Antibodies in the Four Subclasses of IgG by ELISA

JULIA A. GIBSON

Department of Microbiology, Cardiothoracic Institute, Brompton Hospital, Fulham Road, London SW3 6HP

Introduction

Antibody structure and function

All antibodies are thought to have evolved from a single prototype IgM immunoglobulin chain of 110 amino acids. Duplication and mutation of the genes encoding this primitive molecule have produced the five classes now known, i.e. IgM, IgG, IgA, IgE and IgD. An antibody molecule is made up of a pair of identical heavy (long) chains and a pair of identical light (short) chains (Fig. 1). The light chains come in two forms: kappa and lambda, κ and λ, which are not related to antibody class. They have two domains, one variable (V_L) and one constant (C_L). The heavy chains also have one variable domain (V_H) and, in the case of IgM, four constant domains (C_H). The variable regions on one heavy and one light chain form one of the two antigen-combining sites i.e. they give the idiotype (antigen specificity) of the antibody. The amino acid sequences of the constant region characterize antibody class and result in different physiological functions (Table 1). It is thought that IgG derives from IgM through the loss of the C $\mu2$ domain, and IgA similarly by loss of C $\mu3$. IgD also has only three C_H domains. The chains are linked by disulphide bonds, which occur in different positions in all the classes.

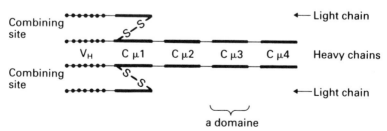

FIG. 1. The structure of IgM.

Immunological Techniques
in Microbiology

TABLE 1. *Characteristics of the five antibody classes*

Characteristic	IgM	IgG	IgA	IgE	IgD
% of total Ig in normal human serum:	8%	74%	17%	<1%	1%
Form:	Pentamer	Monomer	Dimer	Monomer	Monomer
Mainly found in:	Blood stream	Tissue	Seromucous secretions	Blood	Blood
Activities:	Agglutination Cytolysis Opsonization	Neutralization Opsonization Cytolysis	? Prevention of bacterial adherence	Rejection of metazoan parasites (gut) Degranulation of mast cells (allergy)	? Influence of lymphocyte function
Complement fixation:	Yes	Yes	Alternative pathway	No	No
Remarks:	1° response	Predominant Crosses placenta	Locally produced		Found on surface of B lymphocytes

Subclasses have been described for IgG and IgA (Linde *et al.*, 1983). These are due to variations of not more than 10% in the amino acid sequences of the heavy chains. The prevalence and functional characteristics of the IgG subclasses are shown in Table 2.

The combination of antibodies produced in an immune response varies according to the host's genetic make-up, the chemistry and dose of the antigen, and history of previous exposure.

The genetic traits which control or restrict an individual's response are of two kinds: (1) the immune response (Ir) region of the major histocompatibility complex

TABLE 2. *Properties of the subclasses of IgG*

Characteristic	Subclasses of IgG			
	IgG1	IgG2	IgG3	IgG4
% total IgG in normal human serum	65%	23%	8%	4%
Electrophoretic mobility	Slow	Slow	Slow	Fast
Spontaneous agglutination	−	−	+ + +	−
Gm allotypes	Gm(1) (2) (3) (17)	Gm (23)	Gm (5) (6) (10) (11) (13–16) (21) (24) (26) (27)	None known
Ga site reacting with rheumatoid factor	+ + +	+ + +	−	+ + +
Protein A binding	+ + +	+ + +	−	+ + +
Complement fixation (classical pathway)	+ + +	+ +	+ + + +	±
Binding to monocytes	+ + +	+	+ + +	±
Binding to heterologous skin	+ +	−	+ +	+ +
Blocking IgE binding	−	−	−	+
Crossing the placenta	+ +	±	+ +	+ +
Antibody dominance	Anti-Rh	Anti-dextran Anti-levan	Anti-Rh	Anti-Factor VIII

codes for a glycoprotein (Ia) antigen on cell surfaces which appears to affect cooperative interactions between cells involved in cell-mediated immunity and antibody production; and (2) the allotypic determinants in the constant regions of the antibodies. The Ir genes dictate whether or not a particular antigen can be recognized, and the allotype may control the subclass of IgG which is produced if a response is made.

The classes of antibodies found in infection generally follow a common pattern: the first circulating antibodies are IgM, with IgG antibodies increasing as the IgM response fades (at about 1 week) and reaching larger proportions. If the seromucous membranes are involved in the disease (gut, lung or genito-urinary tract) IgA will be produced locally and some finds its way into the blood stream. Antibodies in the IgE class are involved in immune reactions against helminths and are also responsible for allergic reactions, although the factors governing when and why certain individuals become allergic are not well understood. IgD has been relatively recently recognized and its role is not yet clear.

Within the framework of genetics and class indicated above, the chemical nature and the dose of an antigen may dictate the subclass of antibody it stimulates. A variety of investigations have indicated that:

1 IgG1 is generally stimulated by proteins. Measles, CMV and tetanus toxoid antibodies are predominantly of this subclass.
2 IgG2 results from stimulation with polysaccharides.
3 IgG3 is the predominant antibody against polio and herpes simplex viruses.
4 IgG4 levels are raised in severe cases of grass pollen allergy.
5 IgA1 predominates in saliva following challenge with streptococcal protein, carbohydrate or dextran whereas IgA2 predominates in saliva following streptococcal lipopolysaccharide challenge.

This great diversity in antibody responses must be explored if we are to use antibody assays to their best effect. A class-specific enzyme assay for IgG using a polyclonal conjugate may be more efficient at detecting the major subclass (IgG1) than the other subclasses. A serum containing substantial levels of antibody in subclasses other than IgG1 may therefore give a misleading result.

Enzyme-linked assays may easily be adapted to test for any class or subclass of antibody by altering the specificity of the conjugate. We suggest that assays for antibodies in the subclass of IgG may be of value for the following reasons:

1 To define more accurately the humoral immune response.
2 To provide a more sensitive diagnostic test.
3 To examine individual variations in antibody response.
4 To discover whether a particular type of antibody is more protective than others.
5 To look for antibody patterns of a prognostic value in chronic disease.

ELISA

The assay for specific antibodies in the four subclasses of IgG is represented in Fig. 2. Antigen absorbs non-specifically by hydrophobic forces to the plastic of a microtitre plate and succeeding reagents attach specifically, so that the amount of enzyme in a well is proportional to the concentration of specific antibodies in the subclass under test. This enzyme is detected by an appropriate substrate which gives a visible change.

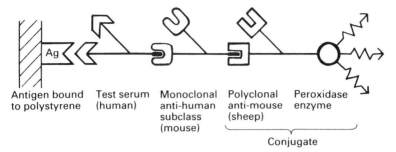

Antigen bound   Test serum   Monoclonal   Polyclonal   Peroxidase
to polystyrene   (human)   anti-human   anti-mouse   enzyme
                               subclass   (sheep)
                               (mouse)   ╰──────────────────────╯
                                                    Conjugate

FIG. 2.   ELISA for specific antibodies in the four subclasses of IgG (schematic representation).

The advantages of using ELISA are:

1 It is very sensitive and may be made very specific.
2 It does not depend on the biological function of the antibody (in contrast to complement fixing, haemagglutination and neutralization tests).
3 Large numbers of tests may be done simultaneously.
4 It uses small quantities of reagents and is therefore relatively cheap.
5 The substrate can be chosen according to the available instrumentation.
6 The flexibility of the test allows it to be adapted to almost any situation.

For reviews of the technique see Herrman (1986), Kurstak (1985), van Weemen (1985) and Yolken (1986).

The components of the test: general considerations
(Suppliers are listed in Appendix III.)

Assay plates

Disposable, flat bottomed 96 well microtitre trays are used. These are manufactured by several companies in rigid polystyrene (Alpha, Becton–Dickinson, Dynatech, Flow, Nunc, Sterilin) and flexible polyvinylchloride (PVC) (Becton–Dickinson, Dynatech, Flow). The polystyrene plates may be specially processed for use in ELISA (Flow Laboratories and Nunc). Dynatech also manufacture plates in Immulon plastic specifically for ELISA.

Polystyrene plates are normally more suitable than PVC because the binding capacity of polystyrene is greater for most antigens. Since the binding to plastic varies with the chemistry of the antigen it is essential to test a variety of plates to find the most suitable for a specific antigen. It is possible that, in a complex antigenic preparation such as a bacterial sonicate, different fractions will adhere to different plates. As the antibody response in each subclass may be directed to specific fractions of the antigen, more than one type of plate may be needed when testing for the four subclasses of IgG.

It is also necessary to test the plates for uniformity of antigen adherence in all wells. The treatments mentioned above are designed to improve this property, which can otherwise be a major source of experimental error.

There are alternative systems available, where the antigen is fixed to a transferable solid phase. Plastic beads (Northumbria Biologicals) are said to provide a particularly uniform surface for antigen attachment, and can be magnetized for easy removal from the wells of a plate, or from tubes (see the chapter by C. J. Stannard et al., pp. 59–72). A plate with plastic pins in the same conformation as a microtitre plate (Nunc) is useful for assay of monoclonal antibody production without disturbing the cultures.

Antigen

The requirement for antigen purity depends on the purpose of the test. In measuring mycobacterial antibodies a crude ultrasonicate of organisms gives better results than a purified antigen because people respond in varying degrees to different epitopes. In other diseases a crude antigen may give cross-reactions which obscure the results, and it may be necessary to extract a specific fraction by chemical or immunological methods. Most proteins adhere easily by passive hydrophobic bonding to plastic. In some cases lyophilization may improve the adherence (Rote et al., 1980). Polysaccharides adhere less easily, and cyanogen bromide may be used to bind them actively to paper (Papierniak et al., 1982). Glycolipids do not adhere by passive bonding but may be attached to microplates by adding sodium desoxycholate to the buffer (Reggiardo & Middlebrook, 1974). It is evident, therefore, that when using a mixed antigen for passive coating there is a tendency for proteins to be selectively retained.

Buffers

A number of buffer systems are in use. Generally the antigen is coated in an alkaline carbonate buffer approximately 0.1 M, pH 9.5–9.8. There must be absolutely no detergent in this buffer.

For subsequent washes and dilutions, phosphate buffered saline pH 7.2–7.4 is used with the addition of a blocking agent or detergent to reduce any further non-specific binding of reagents to the plate or previously bound reagents. Tween 20 at 0.05% is the most usual, and bovine serum albumin (BSA) may be used on its own at 0.5% or in combination with Tween.

The buffer used when adding substrate is chosen to maximise enzyme activity. When the enzyme is alkaline phosphatase, a sodium carbonate buffer 0.05 M, pH 9.8, with or without 0.001 M magnesium chloride, is used. An alternative is 0.1 M diethanolamine at the same pH.

For peroxidase conjugates a citrate buffer 0.05 M, pH 4, is often used for the substrate buffer.

Sodium azide (0.02%) can be added as a preservative for buffers prior to the substrate buffer when the enzyme is alkaline phosphatase. It must not be used with peroxidase as it stops its activity.

Test sera

It is important to store sera at $-20\ ^{\circ}C$ or lower before use and to avoid repeated freezing and thawing which reduces the antibody titre.

Sera are usually tested at the dilution of $1/100$–$1/200$. If neat serum is tested the prozone phenomenon may cause false low readings.

Anti-subclass sera

There are a number of sera commercially available, both monoclonal and polyclonal, usually raised in sheep (Janssen, Miles Scientific, Serotec). In some systems, absorption with antigen may be required even with monoclonal antibodies.

Conjugates

A monoclonal anti-species antibody does not always bind effectively to a monoclonal anti-subclass antibody, and so it is recommended that a polyclonal anti-species conjugate is used to detect the anti-subclass antibodies. Many conjugates arc commercially available containing either alkaline phosphatase or horseradish peroxidase (Janssen, Miles Scientific, Serotec, Seralab, Unipath). They can be made in the laboratory quite successfully if the antiserum for conjugation is of high purity and high titre (e.g. Dako Ltd). Most conjugates are formed by a chemical oxidation–reduction reaction. A gentler method, preserving higher enzyme activity, is to couple biotin (part of the vitamin B coenzyme complex) to both antibody and enzyme. These are then mixed with avidin (extracted from egg albumin). This substance has a very high natural affinity for biotin and in linking with it creates the antibody–enzyme conjugate (see the chapter by G. Coghill et al., pp. 87–110).

Substrates

A variety of substrates have been used for peroxidase enzyme (Al-Kaissi & Mostratos, 1983; Saunders, 1979). When making a choice, possible carcinogenicity and stability of the coloured product should be considered. The enzymic action may be stopped by the addition of strong acid (for peroxidase) or strong alkali (for alkaline phosphatase) but some spontaneous colour development often persists. All colour reactions should proceed in the dark and plates should be kept dark if not read immediately.

An amplified colour reaction can be obtained using an NADH-NAD cycle to mediate the continuous conversion of a colourless tetrazolium salt to a coloured product. This amplification is said to give a more sensitive system as well as a faster result (Johannson *et al.*, 1986).

Recently, an enzyme-linked fluorescent assay (ELFA) has been described. This compares favourably with standard ELISA for sensitivity and gives a fluorescence which is stable and unaffected by light (Dave *et al.*, 1986).

The commonly-used substrates and their methods of use are shown in Table 3.

Controls

All reagents must be tested for non-specific reactivity. Every combination should be tested with substrate on each plate so that problems can be instantly pinpointed. The full set of reagent controls required is:

1 Antigen.
2 Anti-subclass monoclonal antibody (MAb).
3 Conjugate.
4 Antigen with MAb.
5 Antigen with conjugate.
6 MAb with conjugate.
7 Antigen, MAb and conjugate.
8 Test serum with antigen and conjugate (no MAb).

The reproducibility of the test is better if the outer wells of a plate are not used for test sera because the readings tend to be higher here than elsewhere, possibly because of evaporation.

Reading the test

For some 'yes/no' type of tests visual interpretation of the plates may be possible. Usually an automatic plate reader with or without a computerized integrator and printer is used (Dynatech Laboratories, Flow Laboratories, Perkin–Elmer, Wellcome Diagnostics). These give quick and reliable results when the optical quality of the plates is consistent.

Standardization of results

ELISA is notoriously variable from day to day and from plate to plate. Even in carefully controlled experimental conditions there are variations between plates in a single test batch. In order to overcome this difficulty all tests should be done in duplicate, and a standard serum (or serum pool) of high titre must be included in every plate: the test readings being expressed as a ratio of the standard. The standard itself is given an arbitrary value, e.g. 1.0 absorbance units.

A refinement of this calculation is to plot a dilution curve for the standard serum and calculate other values from it by the method of least squares. Since the

TABLE 3. *Enzyme substrates and methods of use*

Enzyme	Substrate*	Buffer	Stop	Colour	Read at	Remarks
Peroxidase	ABTS (0.05%) + H_2O_2 (0.003%)	Citrate/phosphate (0.05 mM, pH 4)	HF or NaF (0.1 M) (0.08 M)	Blue	414 nm	Low grade mutagen
	ASA (0.1%) + H_2O_2 (0.003%)	Phosphate/EDTA (10 mM/0.1 mM, pH 5.6)		Brown	492 nm	Limited solubility
	OPD (0.2% + H_2O_2 (0.003%)	Citrate/phosphate (0.1 M, pH 4.5)	HCl (1 M)	Orange	490 nm	Irritant Mutagenic
		or				
		Methanol (50%)	H_2SO_4 (2.5 M)			
	TMB (0.005%) + H_2O_2 (0.003%)	Acetate + Nitroferrocyanide (10 mM pH 3.3) (0.1%)	H_2SO_4	Yellow	450 nm	Non-toxic
	PHPA (0.37%)	Tris-HCl (0.05 M, pH 7.8)	–	Fluorescent	ex 316 emit 414	Very stable
Alkaline phosphatase	NPP (0.1%)	Sodium carbonate + $MgCl_2$ (0.05 M, pH 9.8) (10 mM)	NaOH (1 M)	Yellow	400 nm	Non-toxic
		or				
		Diethanolamine + $MgCl_2$ (1 M, pH 9.8) (0.5 mM)	NaOH (3 M)			
		or				
		Glycine + $MgCl_2$ (0.05 M, pH 10.5) (1.5 mM)				

* ABTS = 2,2'—azino—bis (3-ethyl benzthiazoline sulphonic acid). ASA = p-amino salicylic acid (= PAS). OPD = O-phenylenediamine. TMB = 3,3',5,5' tetramethyl-benzidine. PHPA = p-hydroxyphenyl acetic acid. pNPP = p'—nitrophenyl phosphate.

dilution curve is fairly straight and it will not be identical for all sera, due to their differing affinities and avidities, this method is only slightly more accurate than the first, simple ratio method.

Interpretation of results

The significance of a result is judged against the levels of antibody found in a control population from the same geographical area, matched as nearly as possible for age, sex etc., to the sample population. It is necessary to establish a 'cut-off' value to distinguish 'positive' from 'negative' results. This may be:

1 The upper limit of normal (ULN). The highest value found in the control population is taken as the cut-off point above which results are positive and below which they are negative. This gives a test with 100% specificity but, depending on the distribution of the results, may give low sensitivity (i.e. a significant proportion of 'positive' tests are reported as negative).
2 Similar to the method above, the cut-off point can be chosen so that, for example, 95% of controls are below it. This reduces the specificity of the test by 5% but may increase the sensitivity by a much greater percentage (i.e. a greater proportion of 'positive' tests are reported as such).
3 The mean $+2$ standard deviations. This usually includes 97.5% of 'normal' values and is suitable if the data are parametrically distributed.

The results may be expressed as the optical density read-outs, but, as discussed above, these fluctuate from test to test, unless they are corrected against the control readings. An alternative is to express results as a percentage of that of a known strongly positive control serum. A technique that we have found useful is the expression of results as multiples of the mean of the control sera readings from healthy individuals, which is assigned a value of 1. This, the calculation of the Multiple of Adult Norm (MAN), has the advantage that it is unaffected by changes in experimental conditions.

Materials and methods

Preparation of peroxidase conjugate

Materials:

> Polyclonal antiserum to species of monoclonal anti-subclass sera.
> Horseradish peroxidase (HRP) type VI (Sigma Chemical Co. Ltd).
> Polyethylene glycol, molecular weight 8000 (PEG).
> Sodium periodate 0.1 M.
> Sodium borohydride 4% w/v in water.
> Glycerol 60% in sodium borate buffer.

Buffers: Sodium carbonate 0.01 M pH 9.5 (see Appendix II).
         Sodium carbonate 0.20 M pH 9.5.
         Sodium acetate 1 mM pH 4.4.
         Sodium borate 0.15 M pH 7.4.
Dialysis tubing

Method:

1 Centrifuge the serum at 2500 rpm for 15 min to remove any precipitated protein, and decant.

2 Estimate the protein concentration e.g. using Folin–Ciocalteau reagent, see Appendix I.

3 If the serum protein concentration is < 8 mg per ml, reduce the volume by putting the serum in dialysis tubing and covering with solid PEG for 15–60 min.

4 Take the volume of serum containing 8 mg of protein and dilute to 1 ml with 0.01 M sodium carbonate buffer. Dialyse overnight at 4 °C against the same buffer.

5 Meanwhile, dissolve 4 mg of HRP in 1 ml distilled water. Prepare 0.1 M sodium periodate freshly (0.107 g in 5 ml distilled water) and add 0.2 ml of this to the HRP. Stir for 20 min. Dialyse overnight at 4 °C against 1 mM sodium acetate buffer. Next day, check that the pH is still acid.

6 Add 0.2 M sodium carbonate buffer to the HRP in small volumes (20–40 μl) until the pH reaches 9–9.5.

7 Immediately add the antiserum and check the pH and, if it falls below 9, add solid sodium carbonate until it reaches 9–9.5. Stir for 2 h at room temperature.

8 Add 0.1 ml of 4% sodium borohydride to reduce unreacted conjugation sites on the HRP. Stand for 2 h at 4 °C. Dialyse overnight at 4 °C against 0.15 M borate buffer.

9 Add an equal volume of 60% glycerol in 0.15 M sodium borate, as a preservative.

10 Store the conjugate at 4 °C (it is stable for at least 6 months).

Preparation of antigen

Our studies involved the detection of antibodies to mycobacteria but the techniques outlined here could easily be modified for preparation of antigen from fungi or other bacteria.

Materials:

BCG (Glaxo).
Sauton's medium.

Method:

1 Put a generous loopful of BCG on the surface of a litre of Sautons medium.

2 Incubate undisturbed at 35 °C for as many weeks as are required to produce a thick pellicle of bacterial growth.

3 Decant the cultures and filter off the medium through Whatmans No. 1 paper.

4 Scrape the bacterial mass into a pyrex beaker and add an equal (w/v) amount of PBS.

5 Sonicate at 2 for 15 min.

6 Centrifuge at 18 000 g for 1 h to remove cell debris.

7 Store supernatent at − 40 °C.

ELISA (Gibson *et al.*, 1987)

Materials:

Plates: Polystyrene 96 well, Nunc Immunoplate I (Gibco Ltd) for IgG1, 2 and 4; Dynatech M129A for IgG3.

Antigen: BCG ultrasonicate.

Sera: Monoclonal anti-human IgG1 (mouse) Unipath BAM15.
Monoclonal anti-human IgG2 (mouse) Unipath BAM10.
Monoclonal anti-human IgG3 (mouse) Unipath BAM 8.
Monoclonal anti-human IgG4 (mouse) Unipath BAM11.
Polyclonal peroxidase-conjugated anti-mouse IgG (sheep) Serotec AAC 10P.

Test sera: appropriate test and control sera.

Substrate: ABTS (Sigma A-1888: 2,2'-Azinodi-(3-ethyl benzthiazoline sulphonic acid).

Hydrogen peroxide (20 volume).

Sodium fluoride 0.32% in distilled water.

Buffers: coating—sodium carbonate 0.05 M, pH 9.6, detergent-free.
washing ⎱ PBS-Tween (oxoid tablets PBS Dulbecco A, 0.05%
diluting ⎰ Tween 20).
Substrate—Citrate/phosphate 0.05 M pH 4.0.

Method:

1 Dilute the antigen in coating buffer, taking care that all glassware is detergent-free. Add 200 μl to each well as required. Cover and leave at room temperature for 2 h.

2 Wash the plates three times in PBS-Tween, using a handheld semi-automatic washer (Nunc Immuno-Wash) or fully automatic washer (e.g. Flow Laboratories, Wellcome Diagnostics). Empty the wells as completely as possible without scratching the plates.

3 Dilute the test and control sera to 1/200 in PBS-Tween and add 200 μl of each to one control and two test wells. Add 200 μl PBS-Tween to all other wells. Cover and leave at room temperature for 2 h.

4 Wash as before.

5 Dilute monoclonal anti-subclass sera in PBS-Tween and absorb with antigen for 30 min before use (The anti-sera to IgG1–4 required 20 µl, 10 µl, 10 µl and 100 µl per 10 ml of serum dilution respectively). Add 200 µl to each of the appropriate wells. Add 200 µl of PBS-Tween to all other wells. Leave, covered, overnight at room temperature.

6 Wash as before.

7 Dilute the conjugate in PBS-Tween and add antigen for absorption (for IgG1, IgG2 and IgG3 10 µl antigen per 25 ml conjugate. For IgG4, 200 µl per 15 ml conjugate). After 30 min, add 200 µl to each well. Leave covered at room temperature for 2 h.

8 Wash as before.

9 Dissolve 50 mg ABTS in 100 ml of substrate buffer. Just before use, add 20 µl of 20 vol hydrogen peroxide and mix. Add 200 µl substrate to all wells. Protect the plates from light and leave for 1 h at room temperature.

10 Add 50 µl of sodium fluoride solution to every well, taking the same direction and time as was used for the substrate addition. Keep the plates dark.

11 Read the absorbance values of all wells using a 414 nm filter (Flow Multiscan MC).

Titrations required (Fig. 3):

1 *Antigen*: the antigen must be titrated separately for each subclass serum. Take two positive sera and test a full range of antigen dilutions, using the monoclonal serum at two arbitrary dilutions, (e.g. 1/500 and 1/1000) and the conjugate also at two dilutions (e.g. 1/2000 and 1/5000). The serum dilutions may have to be adjusted to obtain a range of readings within the readable scale. Select the highest dilution of antigen which gives a maximum reaction.

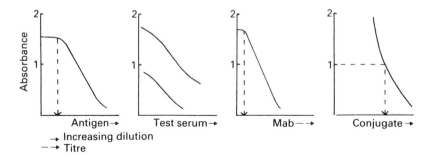

FIG. 3. Titrations for ELISA reagents.

2 *Test sera*: it is customary to test sera at one dilution in the range 1/50–1/200. A titration of one or two positive sera is a useful check on the system once all other dilutions have been worked out: absorbance should be approximately proportional to serum concentration giving a near-straight line graph. If there is an obvious deviation from the straight line graph, results from sera with different levels of antibody will not be directly comparable.

3 *Anti-subclass sera*: these are used at the highest dilution giving maximum reaction unless this dilution gives unacceptably high control readings. The dilution chosen should give maximum differentiation between positive and negative sera. If the anti-subclass sera bind significantly to the antigen in the absence of a positive test serum, they can be absorbed with antigen for 30 min before use. The minimum quantity of antigen needed should be established.

4 *Conjugate*: from the titration curve of the conjugate a dilution giving a reading of approximately 1.0 absorbance units with a strongly positive serum is chosen. Again, absorption with antigen may be required. (In our test the conjugated serum was raised using Freund's complete adjuvant i.e. with mycobacterial antigens, and the resulting mycobacterial antibodies were absorbed out before use.)

Appendix I

Estimation of protein concentration

Reagents

A Sodium carbonate 2% in 0.1 M Sodium hydroxide.
B Sodium citrate 1%, Copper sulphate-$5H_2O$ 0.5% in distilled water.
C 1 ml of B mixed with 50 ml A.
D 10 ml Folin–Ciocalteau reagent mixed with 9.4 ml distilled water.

Method

1 Mix 0.2 ml of standard (Bovine serum albumin, BSA, in steps from 10 µg to 150 µg/ml) or sample with 2 ml of **C**. Stand at room temperature for 10 min.
2 Add 0.2 ml of **D**, mix well and stand for 0.5–2 h.
3 Read absorbance at 750 nm.
4 Draw a standard curve and read test values from it.

Appendix II

Buffer preparations

Method:
Prepare solutions A and B in distilled water.
Add solution A to solution B slowly while stirring, and monitor the pH until it reaches the required value. (The proportion A:B is given as a rough guide only.)

Buffer			A	B	A:B
Sodium carbonate	0.01 M	pH 9.5	Sodium carbonate Na_2CO_3 1.060 g/l	Sodium bicarbonate $NaH CO_3$ 0.840 g/l	1:2
	0.05 M	pH 9.6	Na_2CO_3 5.300 g/l	$NaH CO_3$ 4.200 g/l	1:2
	0.20 M	pH 9.5	Na_2CO_3 21.198 g/l	$NaH CO_3$ 16.802 g/l	1:2
Sodium acetate	1 mM	pH 4.4	Sodium acetate $CH_3 COONa$ 0.082 g/l	Acetic acid $CH_3 COOH$ 0.060 g/l	1:2
Sodium borate	0.15 M	pH 7.4	Di-Sodium tetraborate (Borax) $Na_2B_4O_7.10H_2O$ 1.907 g/50 ml	Boric acid H_3BO_3 6.184 g/l	1:30
Citrate/ phosphate	0.05 M	pH 4.0	Di-Sodium hydrogen ortho-phosphate $Na_2H PO_4.2H_2O$ 8.90 g/l	Citric acid $C_6H_8O_7.H_2O$ 10.500 g/l	2:3

Appendix III

Suppliers

Alpha Laboratories Ltd, 40, Parnham Drive, Eastleigh, Hampshire, SO5 4NU.
Becton Dickinson U.K. Ltd, Between Town Roads, Cowley, Oxford, OX4 3LY.
Dako Ltd, 22, The Arcade, The Octagon, High Wycombe, Bucks, HP11 2HT.
Dynatech Laboratories Ltd, Daux Road, Billingshurst, Sussex, RH14 9SJ.
Flow Laboratories Ltd, Woodstock Hill, Harefield Road, Rickmansworth, Herts, WD3 1PQ.
Gibco Europe Ltd, PO Box 35, Trident House, Renfrew Road, Paisley, PA3 4EF.
Glaxo Laboratories Ltd, Greenford Road, Greenford, Middlesex, UB6 0HE.
Janssen Life Sciences Products, Grove, Wantage, Oxon, OX12 0DQ.
Miles Scientific, PO Box 37, Stoke Poges, Slough, SL2 4LY.
Northumbria Biologicals Ltd, South Nelson Industrial Estate, Cramlington, Northumberland, NE22 9HL.
Nunc—See Gibco Europe Ltd.
Oxoid Ltd, Wade Road, Basingstoke, Hampshire, RG24 0PW.

Perkin-Elmer Ltd, Post Office Lane, Beaconsfield, Bucks, HP9 1QA.
Seralab Ltd, Crawley Down, Sussex, RH10 4FF.
Serotec Ltd, Unit 22, Bankside, Station Field Industrial Estate, Kidlington, Oxford, OX5 1JD.
Sigma Chemical Co. Ltd, Fancy Road, Poole, Dorset, BH7 7NH.
Sterilin Ltd, Clockhouse Lane, Feltham, Middlesex, TW14 8QS.
Unipath Ltd, Norse Road, Bedford, MK41 0GQ.
Wellcome Diagnostics, Temple Hill, Dartford, DA1 5AH.

References

AL-KAISSI, E. & MOSTRATOS, A. 1983 Assessment of substrates for horseradish peroxidase in enzyme immunoassay. *Journal of Immunological Methods* 58, 127–132.

DAVE, J. R., TAYLOR, P., GRANGE, J. M. & GAYA, H. 1986 A new enzyme-linked fluorescence assay (ELFA) for use with peroxidase-antibody conjugates: a comparison with ELISA for the quantification of IgM antibodies to hepatitis B core antigen. *Journal of Medical Microbiology* 21, 271–274.

GIBSON, J. A., GRANGE, J. M., BECK, J. S. & KARDJITO, T. 1987 Antibody response to *Mycobacterium tuberculosis* in the four subclasses of IgG in patients with smear-positive pulmonary tuberculosis. *European Journal of Respiratory Diseases* 70, 29–34.

HERRMAN, J. E. 1986 Enzyme-linked immunoassays for the detection of microbial antigens and their antibodies (172 references). *Advances in Applied Microbiology* 31, 271–292.

JOHANNSON, A., ELLIS, D. H., BATES, D. L., PLUMP, A. M. & STANLEY, C. J. 1986 Enzyme amplification for immunoassays. Detection limit of one hundredth of an attomole. *Journal of Immunological Methods* 87, 7–11.

KURSTAK, E. 1985 Progress in enzyme immunoassays: production of reagents, experimental design and interpretation (98 references). *Bulletin of the World Health Organization* 63, 793–811.

LINDE, G. A., HAMMARSTROM, L., PERSSON, M. A. A., SMITH, E., SUNDQUVIST, V. A. & WAHREN, B. 1983 Virus-specific antibody activity of different subclasses of IgG and IgA in cytomegalo infections. *Infection and Immunology* 42, 237–244.

PAPIERNIAK, C. K., KLEGERMAN, M. E., BOYER, K. M., KRETSCHMER, R. R. & GOTOFF, S. P. 1982 An enzyme-linked immunosorbent assay (ELISA) for human IgG antibody to the type Ia polysaccharide of group B streptococcus. *Journal of Laboratory and Clinical Medicine* 100, 385–398.

REGGIARDO, Z. & MIDDLEBROOK, G. 1974 Serologically active glycolipid families from *Mycobacterium bovis* BCG. *American Journal of Epidemiology* 100, 469–476.

ROTE, N. S., TAYLOR, N. L., SHIGEOKA, A. O., SCOTT, J. R. & HILL, H. R. 1980 Enzyme-linked immunoassay (ELISA) for group B streptococcal antigens. *Infection and Immunity* 27, 118–123.

SAUNDERS, G. C. 1979 The art of solid-phase enzyme immunoassay including protocols. In *Immunoassays in the clinical laboratory* ed. Nakamura, R. M., Dick, W. R. & Tucker, G. S. Vol 3 in the series *Laboratory and research methods in Biology & Medicine* pp. 99–118. New York: Alan R. Liss Inc.

VAN WEEMEN, B. K. 1985 ELISA: Highlights of the present state of the art. *Journal of Urological Methods* 10, 371–378.

YOLKEN, R. H. 1986 Enzyme immunoassay for the detection of microbial antigens and prospects for improved assays. *Yale Journal of Biology and Medicine* 59, 24–31.

ELISA for the Detection of Total Serum IgE: Speed and Sensitivity

D. M. KEMENY AND D. RICHARDS

Department of Medicine, United Medical and Dental Schools, Guy's Hospital, St Thomas' Street, London SE1 9RT

Introduction

The sensitivity and speed of immunoassays are controlled by the affinity of the immune reaction, the medium in which it is carried out and the signal used to monitor it. The use of radioisotopes (Yalow & Berson, 1960) greatly increased the sensitivity of immunoassays and when these are carried out with antigen or antibody bound to a solid-phase, it is possible to increase the concentration of reagents used and so drive the assay to give greater sensitivity and speed as envisaged by Miles & Hales (1968). In the field of allergy, where small quantities of reaginic antibody (IgE) can be sufficient to sensitize tissues, these techniques have proved invaluable and assays for total and specific IgE are among the most sensitive developed (Wide & Porath, 1966; Wide *et al.*, 1967; Ceska & Lundkvist, 1972; Ceska *et al.*, 1972). The advantages of solid-phase immunometric assays have, perhaps, been best realized in ELISA (Engvall & Perlmann 1971) where the use of plastic, with its low non-specific protein binding characteristics, permits high concentrations of reagents to be used. As labels, enzymes offer a potential for greater sensitivity, compared with radioisotopes, because of the inherent amplification of signal that they provide (one molecule of enzyme generates many molecules of product). This amplification can be further increased by using radiolabelled substrates (ultrasensitive enzymatic radioimmunoassays) (Harris *et al.*, 1979; Hsu *et al.*, 1980) or second enzymes that are activated by the product of the first (Lowry *et al.*, 1961; Fenerly & Walker, 1965; Self, 1985; Johanssonn *et al.*, 1986).

A further development in immunology has increased the potential of immunoassays. The discovery that fusion of antibody secreting plasma cells with myeloma cell lines could lead to clones of antibody producing cells with identical specificity (monoclonal) made it possible to tailor the antibody to the specific test used. In this report we describe the use of high affinity mouse monoclonal antibody

Immunological Techniques
in Microbiology

to human IgE as a capture antibody, and alkaline phosphatase labelled rabbit anti-IgE (AP anti-IgE) as a detection reagent. The various parameters that affect the performance of the assay are discussed.

Materials and Methods

Reagents and sera

Reagents

Immulon (M 129/A) and immuno-1 (Nunc) microtitre plates were purchased from Dynatech Ltd, (U.K.) and Gibco Ltd (U.K.) respectively. Normal rabbit serum was purchased from Sera Lab Ltd (England). Tween 20, alkaline phosphatase (EC 3.1.3.1) and *p*-nitrophenyl phosphate were purchased from Sigma Ltd (U.K.). All other reagents were purchased from BDH Ltd (U.K.).

Antigens and antisera

Mouse monoclonal anti-IgE (clone 7.12) which had an affinity of 9×10^{-10} was a kind gift from Professor A. Saxon, UCLA, U.S.A. (Saxon *et al.*, 1980). Rabbit anti-human IgE was prepared by immunization of New Zealand white rabbits with 0.25 mg IgE myeloma (PS) protein, in complete Freunds Adjuvant into the foot pads and boosted with 0.25 mg in incomplete Freunds Adjuvant subcutaneously at 2 weekly intervals for 8 weeks. The rabbit anti-IgE was absorbed twice over human IgG (Karbi Ltd, Sweden), bound to Sepharose 4B (Pharmacia plc, U.K.) (10 mg IgG/ml of gel) and with normal human serum-coated Sepharose (10 ml serum per ml of gel). The absorbed antibody gave no precipitin lines by double gel diffusion against any immunoglobulin other than IgE. The affinity purification of this antibody was carried out using 1 ml of Sepharose coated with 10 mg of IgE myeloma WT (WT serum was a kind gift from Dr D. R. Stanworth, Birmingham University, U.K.), and 5 mg of purified anti-IgE was coupled to 5 mg of alkaline phosphatase using the single step gluteraldehyde procedure (Avrameas *et al.*, 1978). The antibody–enzyme conjugate was stored in a Tris/HCl buffer 0.5 M, pH 8.0 containing containing 50% glycerol and 1% bovine serum albumin at 4 °C.

Serum samples

IgE myeloma (WT) serum which contained 50 mg/ml of IgE was used to optimise the assay. In the experiments in which the performance of the developed assay is shown, IgE reference samples were taken from the Phadebas IgE RIA kit (Pharmacia).

ELISA

All incubation volumes were of 100 μl and all incubation buffers contained indicator solution to make it easier to see which wells had been filled. This comprized 0.5% v/v phenol red (60 mg/100 ml H_2O) and 0.5% v/v napthalene or amido black (40 mg/100 ml H_2O), and imparts a lilac colour to the buffer at alkaline pH and a green colour at neutral pH. Its use was kindly suggested by Dr R. C. Aalberse, Red Cross, Amsterdam, Holland.

In the experiments in which the sample and the enzyme-labelled anti-IgE were added simultaneously, the sample was coloured with the amido black solution (Blue) and the AP anti-IgE with the phenol red solution (Red). The coating buffer was carbonate/bicarbonate, 0.1 M, pH 9.6, and the assay buffer was phosphate buffered saline (PBS), 0.05 M, pH 7.4, containing 0.001% w/v sodium azide, 1% normal rabbit serum and 0.5% Tween 20. The assay procedure was as follows:

Rapid assay (20 min)

Microtitre plates were coated with 1 μg/ml monoclonal anti-IgE at 4 °C overnight in coating buffer. The plate was washed three times with PBS containing Tween 20, 0.005% (wash solution) and the sample diluted in assay buffer was added and immediately followed by the enzyme-labelled anti-IgE (1/50, approximately 40 μg/ml). After 10 min the plate was washed twice with wash solution and once with distilled water. The substrate, p-nitrophenyl phosphate 1.0 mg/ml in pH 9.8 diethanolamine buffer, 0.1 M) was then added and, following a 10 min incubation, the reaction was stopped by the addition of 50 μl of 3 M NaOH and the optical density was read on a Titertek Multiskan (Flow Ltd, U.K.) microtitre plate reader at 405 nm.

Sensitive assay (8 h)

This was carried out as for the rapid assay with the following modifications. The sample was incubated for 3 h at 4 °C with the monoclonal anti-IgE coated plate. The enzyme-labelled anti-IgE was added after washing the plate three times and was at a 1/500 dilution (4 μg/ml). The substrate was incubated with the plate for 90 min at 37 °C. The intra-assay coefficient of variation of 12 assays was 6.1%.

Statistical analysis

The correlation between the RIA and ELISA was carried out by linear regression on a BBC model B computer (Acorn Ltd, England) using the BSTAT + statistics programme (Finersoft © 1984).

Results

Optimization of the assay

Every aspect of the test was investigated and our results are summarized here. Two different types of microtitre plate were used: Dynatech M129/A and Nunc immuno-1. Although from different manufacturers, these represented moderate and high capacity plastic respectively and plates from other manufacturers could be expected to perform in a similar fashion—the high capacity plates having been irradiated by the manufacturer. Using different concentrations of mouse monoclonal anti-IgE, their capacity for IgE was tested using myeloma IgE (WT) spiked with I^{125} IgE (Phadebas RIA Ltd, Pharmacia). At concentrations of monoclonal anti-IgE > 1 µg/ml the capacity for IgE was not increased. The high capacity plates, however, bound significantly more IgE (90% up to 100 ng/ml) compared with the moderate capacity plates (56% of IgE bound). This was reflected in the assay and the higher capacity plates gave superior results. The efficiency with which the monoclonal anti-IgE-coated plates bound IgE was so high that it is unlikely that this could be a limiting factor in the assay. Furthermore, binding the monoclonal anti-IgE to the plate with rabbit anti-mouse antibody did not increase its ability to bind IgE although it did reduce the amount of monoclonal antibody required, tenfold.

The enzyme-labelled anti-IgE used proved to be critical. We compared a number of commercially available anti-IgE reagents produced by Sigma, Dako, Boehring and Pharmacia. All performed adequately for routine purposes but the background binding of the first two was too high for maximum sensitivity. The enzyme-labelled anti-IgE prepared in our own laboratory performed as well as the Boehring and Pharmacia products. For all of these antisera the concentration used was important. At high concentrations (Fig. 1), 1/50–1/500 $(40-4$ µg/ml) there was little difference in the colour developed once background binding had been taken into account. Below this concentration the results were poor and although the background binding was low, there was too little enzyme-labelled anti-IgE bound. Whether this is due to the poor performance of such small amounts of bound enzyme is not clear but it is a variable phenomenon that we have observed with some antisera and not with others. It is possible that such variation reflects the degree of denaturation or aggregation of the antibody during the enzyme coupling procedure.

Binding kinetics

The rate at which the sample (IgE) bound to the antibody-coated plates was studied. Maximum binding was reached within 3 h (Fig. 2). The rate of binding was similar

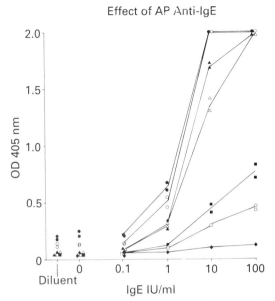

FIG. 1. The effect of the concentration of alkaline–phosphatase labelled rabbit anti-IgE on the assay showing that similar results were obtained at high (●, 1/50; ○, 1/100; ▲, 1/200; △, 1/500) but not low (■, 1/1000; □, 1/2000; ◆, 1/5000) AP anti-IgE concentrations.

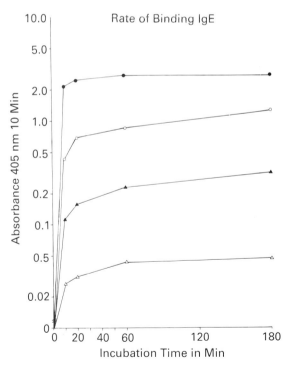

FIG. 2. The rate of binding of IgE to the monoclonal anti-IgE-coated plate was near maximal within 3 h. The rate of binding was higher at 1000 (●) than at 100 (○), 10 (▲) or 1 (△) IU/ml of IgE. AP anti-IgE was used at 1/50 dilution.

for different concentrations of IgE except the highest (1000 IU/ml) which bound
faster (Fig. 3). This is presumably due to the limited capacity of the plates which
were more rapidly saturated by the high concentrations of IgE used. As for IgE,
maximal binding of the enzyme-labelled anti-IgE occurred within 3 h (Fig. 4).
Indeed, at 1/50 near maximal binding occurred in one hour, while at 1/500 this
took longer (Fig. 5). The binding of both IgE and enzyme-labelled anti-IgE was
faster at higher temperatures (Fig. 6).

Assay amplification

Because the monoclonal anti-IgE only recognizes a single epitope on each heavy
chain of the IgE molecule, it seemed likely that there would be little competition
between the monoclonal antibody and the enzyme-labelled anti-IgE for binding to
IgE. Accordingly the assay was simplified by the simultaneous addition of IgE and
enzyme-labelled anti-IgE. The results, using a 1/500 dilution of the alkaline

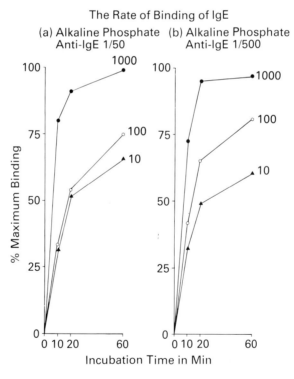

Fig. 3.   The concentration of enzyme-labelled anti-IgE had little affect on the detection of IgE, ●,
1000; ○, 100; or ▲, 10 IU/ml, bound at different time intervals.

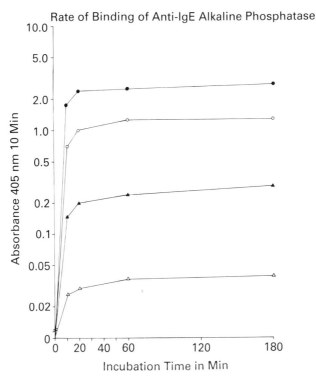

FIG. 4. Binding rate of enzyme-labelled anti-IgE at 1/50 dilution was near maximal at 1 h and was largely independent of the concentration of IgE added (●, 1000; ○, 100; ▲, 10; △, 1 IU/ml IgE).

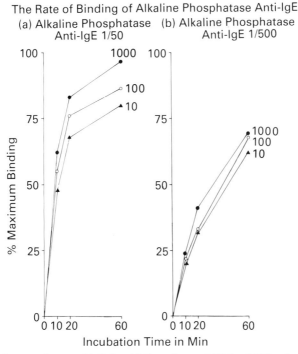

FIG. 5. Binding rate of enzyme labelled anti-IgE was faster at 1/50 than 1/500 and was independent of the concentration of IgE (●, 1000; ○, 100; ▲, 10 IU/ml).

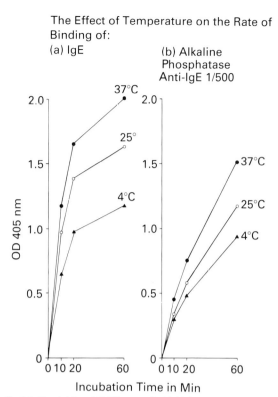

The Effect of Temperature on the Rate of Binding of:

(a) IgE   (b) Alkaline Phosphatase Anti-IgE 1/500

FIG. 6.   Binding of both IgE and AP anti-IgE increased with higher temperatures.

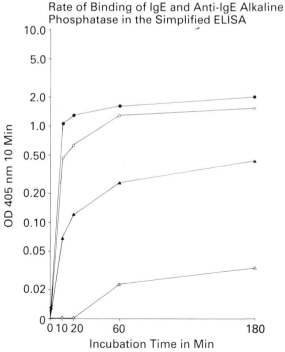

Rate of Binding of IgE and Anti-IgE Alkaline Phosphatase in the Simplified ELISA

FIG. 7.   Simultaneous addition of IgE and enzyme-labelled anti-IgE in a simplified assay procedure gave similar results at 1000 (●), 100 (○) and 10 (▲) IU/ml but slower binding at 1 IU/ml (△).

phosphatase anti-IgE, are shown in Fig. 7. Above 1 IU/ml of IgE similar results were obtained in comparison with the sequential assay procedure. Using this simplified assay it is possible to detect as little as 5 IU/ml of IgE (Fig. 8) in a 20 min assay. Longer sample and substrate incubation increases sensitivity but the major limiting factor is the length of substrate incubation. An enzyme with a faster turnover rate, such as horseradish peroxidase, or amplification using second enzymes (Self, 1985) might be expected to shorten this.

Discussion

In this study we have investigated the different parameters that affect the performance of an assay for human IgE. Using optimal conditions, we found that a high affinity mouse monoclonal anti-IgE (Saxon *et al.*, 1980) was able to bind IgE in

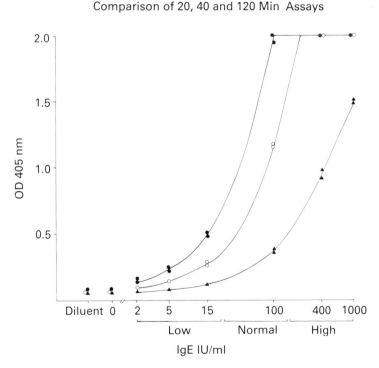

FIG. 8. Comparison of the simplified assay procedure at 20 (▲), 40 (○) and 120 (●) min. The shorter assay time is still able to clearly distinguish low (<20 IU/ml), normal (20–150 IU/ml) and high (>150 IU/ml) IgE levels.

a dose-dependant fashion very rapidly. Furthermore, because the monoclonal anti-IgE only recognizes a single epitope on each IgE heavy chain, there is little interference with the AP anti-IgE. Thus it was possible to use simultaneous addition of IgE and a high concentration of alkaline phosphatase labelled anti-human IgE. Using this simplified assay procedure it was possible to discriminate clinically relevant IgE levels within 20 min. The absolute sensitivity of the method using longer incubation was 0.1 IU/ml of IgE (0.24 ng/ml). The use of a mixture of monoclonal anti-IgE antibodies, clones 7.12 and 4.15 (Saxon *et al.*, 1980) did not enhance the detection of IgE although clone 4.15 on its own performed similarly to 7.12.

We believe that the rapid assay procedure described here would be suitable for determination of IgE levels in the allergy clinic so that information about the likelihood of a patient being atopic would be immediately available. The assay described here is robust, although the rapid procedure is not suitable for multiple determinations due to drifting incubation times across the microtitre plate. Similar procedures could be developed for detection of other analytes provided that the reagents are carefully selected for non-interference and efficacy.

Acknowledgements

Our thanks are due to Mrs P. Powell and Miss C. Langan for typing this manuscript.

References

AVRAMEAS, S., TERNYNCK, T. & GUESDON, J-L. 1978 Coupling of enzymes to antibodies and antigens. *Scandinavian Journal of Immunology* 8, Suppl 7, 7–23.

CESKA, M., ERIKSSON, R. & VARGA, J. M. 1972 Radioimmunosorbent assay of allergens. *Journal of Allergy and Clinical Immunology* 49, 1–9.

CESKA, M. & LUNDKVIST, U. 1972 A new and simple radioimmunoassy method for the determination of IgE. *Immunochemistry* 9, 1021–1030.

ENGVALL, E. & PERLMANN, P. 1971 Enzyme-linked immunosorbent assay (ELISA): quantitative assay of IgG. *Immunochemistry* 8, 871–874.

FENERLY, H. N. & WALKER, P. G. 1965 Kinetic behaviour of calf-intestinal alkaline phosphatase with 4-methyl unbelliferyl phosphate. *Biochemical Journal* 97, 95–103.

HARRIS, C. C., YOLKEN, R. H., KROKAN, H. & HSU, J. C. 1979 Ultrasensitive enzymatic radioimmunoassay: application to detection of cholera toxin and rotavirus. *Proceedings of the National Academy of Science (USA)* 56, 5336–5339.

HSU, I. C., POIRER, M. C., YUSPA, S. H., YOLKEN, R. H. & HARRIS, C. C. 1980 Ultrasensitive enzymatic radioimmunoassay (USEIA) detects femtomoles of acetylaminofluorene—DNA adducts. *Carcinogenesis* 1, 455–458.

JOHANNSSON, A., ELLIS, D. H., BATES, D. L., PLUMB, A. M. & STANLEY, C. J. 1986 Enzyme amplification for immunoassay detection limit of one hundredth of an attomole. *Journal of Immunological Methods* 87, 7–12.

LOWRY, O. H., PARSONEAN, J. U., SCHULTZ, D. W. & ROCK, M. H. 1961 The measurement of pyridine nucleotides by enzymatic cycling. *Journal of Biological Chemistry* **236**, 2746–2755.

MILES, L. E. M. & HALES, C. N. 1968 Labelled antibodies and immunological assay systems. *Nature (London)* **219**, 186–189.

SAXON, A., MORROW, C. & STEVENS, R. H. 1980 Subpopulations of circulating B cells involved in *in vitro* immunoglobulin E production in atopic patients with elevated serum immunoglobulin E. *Journal of Clinical Investigation* **65**, 1457–1468.

SELF, C. H. 1985 Enzyme amplification—a general method applied to provide an immuno assisted assay for placental alkaline phosphatase. *Journal of Immunological Methods* **83**, 389–393.

WIDE, L., BENNICH, H. & JOHANSSON, S. G. O. 1967 Diagnosis of allergy by an *in vitro* test for allergen antibodies. *Lancet* **ii**, 115–117.

WIDE, L. & PORATH, J. 1966 Radioimmunoassay of proteins with the use of Sephadex-coated antibodies. *Biochemica Biophysica Acta* **130**, 257–260.

YALOW, R. S. & BERSON, S. A. 1960 Immunoassay of endogenous plasma insulin in man. *Journal of Clinical Investigation* **39**, 1157–1175.

Magnetic Enzyme Immunoassay (MEIA) for Staphylococcal Enterotoxin B

C. J. STANNARD, P. D. PATEL, S. D. HAINES AND P. A. GIBBS

Leatherhead Food Research Association, Randalls Road, Leatherhead, Surrey KT22 7RY

Introduction

Laboratories investigating outbreaks of staphylococcal food poisoning require rapid and sensitive methods for the detection of staphylococcal enterotoxins in foods. Ingestion of as little as 0.5 µg of staphylococcal enterotoxin can cause symptoms such as vomiting and diarrhoea (Notermans *et al.*, 1983).

Procedures routinely used for the detection and estimation of staphylococcal enterotoxins in foods are complex and lengthy, but have been shown to perform satisfactorily in many laboratories. The procedures normally employed are the extraction of the enterotoxin from the food (2–3 days), followed by the detection of the enterotoxin by the microslide double-immunodiffusion technique (Crowle, 1958), which takes a further 2–3 days. Thus a result could be obtained within a week but frequently takes longer (Holbrook & Baird-Parker, 1975). The sensitivity of this type of technique is 0.1–0.5 µg enterotoxin/100 g food sample (Niskanen, 1977).

Radioimmunoassay (RIA) techniques have been investigated as a more rapid detection method for staphylococcal enterotoxins in foods (Bergdoll & Reiser, 1980). Although RIA methods are highly sensitive and reproducible, providing a result in about 1 day, their routine use is not favoured by the industry because of their dependence on radioisotopes and expensive reagents and instruments.

An alternative to RIA, which obviates the necessity for a radiolabel, is the enzyme immunoassay (EIA). One type of EIA, the enzyme linked immunosorbent assay (ELISA), uses antibody bound to a solid surface to capture the antigen. The solid surface may be plastic beads, the sides of a microtitre well or, in the case of magnetic enzyme immunoassay (MEIA), a magnetic gel. This gel consists of polyacrylamide agarose beads in which iron oxide particles are entrapped, making the separation procedures in the assay simple by use of a magnet. MEIA techniques have been reported for the estimation of immunoglobulins (Guesdon & Avrameas, 1977).

Immunological Techniques
in Microbiology
0–632–01908–5

This chapter describes the development of an MEIA for staphylococcal enterotoxin B and its use for the detection of the toxin in foods.

Principles of MEIA

The principles of the MEIA technique are summarized in Fig. 1. Staphylococcal enterotoxin B antibody is first immobilized on to the magnetic beads. During the assay, if enterotoxin B is present in the sample it will attach to the antibody. Staphylococcal enterotoxin B antibody-conjugated enzyme is then added to the assay vial, and will link to any enterotoxin B that has previously bound to the antibody on the magnetic beads. Unbound antibody-enzyme conjugate is removed. This can be achieved by attracting the magnetic particles to the side or base of the assay vial by using a magnet, and removing the liquid by suction. After washing,

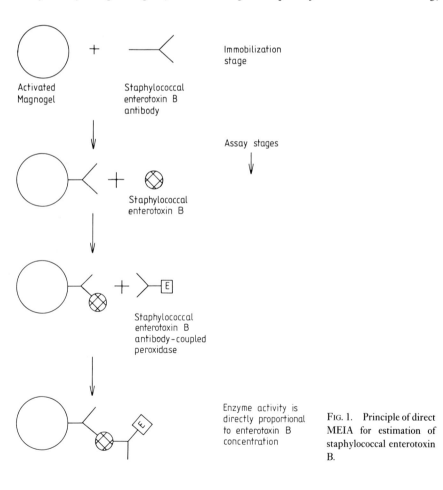

Activated
Magnogel

Staphylococcal
enterotoxin B
antibody

Immobilization
stage

Assay stages

Staphylococcal
enterotoxin B

Staphylococcal
enterotoxin B
antibody-coupled
peroxidase

Enzyme activity is
directly proportional
to enterotoxin B
concentration

Fig. 1. Principle of direct MEIA for estimation of staphylococcal enterotoxin B.

the substrate for the enzyme is added, which will form a coloured product when the enzyme is present. The colour intensity is proportional to the amount of bound enterotoxin. This type of technique is often called a 'sandwich' ELISA, since the enterotoxin is sandwiched between two homologous antibodies.

Experimental Procedure

Materials

Foods

Ham, chicken liver pâté, dried skimmed-milk powder and Cheddar cheese were purchased locally.

Act-Magnogel AcA-44

Act-Magnogel AcA-44 (LKB Ltd, Croydon, Surrey) consists of 4% polyacrylamide and 4% agarose in a bead form with 7% iron oxide (Fe_3O_4) in the matrix, enabling it to be attracted by a magnetic field. The beads are activated by glutaraldehyde and therefore free amino ligands (e.g. in proteins) can be immobilized to the gel.

Staphylococcal enterotoxins and anti-enterotoxin B sera

Staphylococcal enterotoxin B was either purchased (Makor Chemicals Co., Israel) or obtained through the courtesy of Professor M. S. Bergdoll (University of Wisconsin, Madison, U.S.A.). Enterotoxins A, C, D and E were obtained from Serva, Heidelberg. Staphylococcal enterotoxin B antiserum produced in rabbits was either purchased from Makor Chemicals Co. or Serva, or was obtained as a gift from Professor J. Melling (Microbiology Department, CAMR, Porton Down, Wiltshire).

Spicer–Edwards antiserum

A pooled Spicer–Edwards antiserum (Difco) was used as a negative control serum in the MEIA. The antisera consisted of a range of *Salmonella* antiflagellar antibodies and were pooled according to Boothroyd & Baird-Parker (1973). This serum was also used to remove interference with the assay by protein A.

Phosphate-buffered saline-Tween 20 (PBS-Tween)

PBS-Tween (Voller, Bidwell & Bartlett, 1979) consists of NaCl, 8 g; KH_2PO_4, 0.2 g; $Na_2HPO_4.12H_2O$, 2.9 g; KCl, 0.2 g and Tween 20, 0.5 ml in 1 litre of distilled water (pH 7.4).

Horseradish peroxidase and substrate

Horseradish peroxidase was supplied by Sigma (RZ 3.0). The substrate solution consisted of phosphate citrate buffer, pH 5.0 (0.1 M citric acid, 24.3 ml and 0.2 M Na₂HPO₄, 25.7 ml in 50 ml distilled water), into which was dissolved 40 mg orthophenylenediamine (Sigma). Hydrogen peroxide (30% v/v, 40 μl) was added immediately before use.

Methods

Preparation of staphylococcal enterotoxin B serum

Freeze-dried staphylococcal enterotoxin B antiserum (140 mg) was dissolved in 1 ml of 0.5 M phosphate buffer, pH 6.0, and dialysed against approximately 1 litre of the same buffer for 16 h at 4 °C. The dialysed protein was centrifuged (2000 g for 10 min) in order to remove any particulate matter. A sample (50 μl) of the supernatant was mixed with 0.45 ml of 0.04 M phosphate buffer, pH 7.2, containing 0.002% m/v thomerosal and 0.145 M sodium chloride and was used for determining the immunological activity by the double immunodiffusion test (Wood & Payne, 1974). The remaining supernatant was used for coupling to Act-Magnogel AcA-44.

Coupling of staphylococcal enterotoxin B antiserum to Act-Magnogel AcA-44

Act-Magnogel AcA-44 gel (1 ml) was washed twice with about 25 ml of deionized water. After each washing stage the gel was separated from the liquid phase by a magnet (12 × 9 × 42 mm, LKB) and the supernatant was discarded. The gel was then washed twice more with about 25 ml of 0.04 M phosphate buffer, pH 7.2, containing 0.002% m/v thimerosal and 0.145 M sodium chloride. This buffer was used in all subsequent steps unless stated otherwise.

The washed Magnogel was suspended in 0.95 ml of staphylococcal enterotoxin B antiserum and mixed at 4 °C for 16–20 h (RM/54 Rolamix, Luckham Ltd). If clumps of Magnogel were present, either in the initial gel suspension or in any subsequent steps, it was thoroughly vortex-mixed to form a homogeneous suspension.

The antibody-coupled Magnogel was separated by using a magnet, and the supernatant was tested for immunological activity by the double immunodiffusion test (Wood & Payne, 1974). The titre of the residual antiserum was reduced by approximately 3.5-fold after coupling to Magnogel, indicating that most of the immunological activity was bound to the Magnogel.

Purification of anti-enterotoxin IgG antibodies

The purification procedure for anti-enterotoxin IgG antibodies using protein A Sepharose CL-4B gel is described in Appendix I. The purified IgG was then used for coupling to peroxidase.

Coupling of peroxidase to staphylococcal enterotoxin B purified IgG antibodies

The IgG-peroxidase conjugate was prepared as described in Appendix II.

Purification of IgG-peroxidase conjugate by gel permeation chromatography

A column (2.5 × 68 cm) of Ultrogel AcA-34 (LKB Ltd, Surrey) was prepared and equilibrated with 0.1 M phosphate buffer, pH 7.5, containing 0.1 M sodium chloride, according to the procedure described in the instruction manual 'LKB Ultrogel' (1-Z204-E01, 1976).

The conjugate solution (1.5 ml) was applied (flow rate about 0.2 ml/min) and eluted with the equilibration buffer at a flow rate of 0.25 ml/min. The column effluent was continously monitored at 280 nm (for detection of proteins; Uvicord S, LKB) and at 420 nm (SP6-350 Pye-Unicam Spectrophotometer) for detection of horseradish peroxidase; 6 ml fractions were collected.

Fractions comprising peak 2, which contained the conjugate, were pooled and concentrated to dryness by dialysis against 1 litre of 30% w/v polyethylene glycol for 24 h at 4 °C. The dried IgG-peroxidase was resuspended in 1 ml of 0.04 M phosphate-buffered saline containing 0.145 M sodium chloride and 0.002% thimerosal, and was used in the MEIA procedure described later.

Extraction of enterotoxin B from foods

To a 100 g sample of food in a stomacher bag, 1 μg of enterotoxin B and 100 ml (or 150 ml in the case of dried skimmed milk) distilled water were added. Cheese and ham were diced before these additions were made. The food was homogenized in a Colworth 400 Stomacher for 2 min and the slurry was collected in a 250 ml beaker. The slurry was adjusted to pH 4.5 with 6 M hydrochloric acid and then centrifuged at 20 000 g for 20 min at 4 °C (MSE High-Spin 21). The supernatant was collected after passing through a fine-mesh strainer (a tea strainer) and the pH was adjusted to pH 7.5 with 5 M sodium hydroxide. One-quarter volume of chloroform was added and the mixture was stirred vigorously on a magnetic stirrer for about 3 min. The mixture was then centrifuged at 20 000 g for 20 min at 4 °C. Chloroform extraction of the upper aqueous layers was repeated if heavy precipitation was observed. The clear supernatant was decanted and used in the MEIA.

Estimation of enterotoxin B produced by Staphylococcus aureus *in ham*

Staphylococcus aureus NCTC 10654, a known enterotoxin B producer, was inoculated into Trypticase Soy Broth (Gibco) and incubated at 37 °C for 16 h. This culture was diluted 1:10 in sterile quarter-strength Ringer's solution (Oxoid) containing 0.1% w/v Bacteriological Peptone (Difco). One millilitre of this suspension (i.e. about 10[8] colony forming units) was inoculated into 100 g of diced ham, mixed in a stomacher (Colworth Model 400) and incubated at 37 °C for 24 h. Sodium chloride (0.2 M; 100 ml) was then added prior to stomaching and extraction (as above) of the food homogenate.

Similar experiments were done using *Staph. aureus* NCTC 7121 (a non-toxigenic strain which does not produce protein A) and *Staph. aureus* NCTC 8530 (a non-toxigenic strain which produces protein A) to investigate possible interference by protein A.

Estimation of interference by protein A in cheese

One millilitre of solutions of both protein A (1 mg/ml) and enterotoxin B (1 μg/ml) was added to 100 g of cheese and a clear cheese extract was prepared as above. An extract of cheese spiked with enterotoxin B alone was also prepared as a control. These extracts were used in the MEIA for estimation of both enterotoxin B and interference by protein A.

Estimation of staphylococcal enterotoxin B by direct MEIA

The principal features of the assay are shown in Fig. 1. PBS-Tween was used as the diluent throughout this protocol unless specified otherwise.

Wells in a microtitre plate (M129A; Dynatech Laboratories) were washed six times using the Nunc-Immuno-washer 12 system (Gibco). Excess solution was removed by inverting the plate and shaking off the fluid. Standard enterotoxin B solutions (1–100 ng/ml; 100 μl) were added to wells for preparation of a standard curve (in duplicate). For the estimation of enterotoxin B in food extracts, 100 μl of the extract were added to other wells. Negative controls were included using wells containing standard enterotoxin E solutions (0.1–10 μg/ml; 100 μl), wells containing no enterotoxin, and wells containing PBS-Tween only. For the estimation of interference by protein A in cheese, 50 μl of the extracts were reacted with an equal volume of pooled Spicer-Edwards *Salmonella* H antiserum for about 1 h at 37 °C on a Varishaker (speed 5, about 3000 rev/min; Dynatech Laboratories) prior to use in the assay.

To each of the wells, 50 μl of the antibody-coupled Magnogel were added. The plate was covered with a lid (M42R; Dynatech Laboratories) and incubated at 37 °C for 90 min on the Varishaker (speed 5). The Magnogel complex was separated and concentrated at the side of wells by a magnet placed beneath. The liquid phase was then removed by gentle suction with a Pasteur pipette connected to a vacuum source. (*Note*: during this and subsequent stages, it is important to keep the loss of Magnogel to an absolute minimum.) The Magnogel complex was washed three times with PBS-Tween by resuspension of the gel using the Nunc-Immunowasher 12 system without its suction mechanism and repetition of the separation using a magnet as described above.

To each well, 150 µl of the IgG-peroxidase conjugate (1:5000 dilution) was added and the plate was incubated on the Varishaker (speed 5) at 37 °C for 90 min. The Magnogel complex was washed three times as described previously.

To each well, 200 µl of the peroxidase substrate solution was added and the plate was incubated at ambient temperature for 30 min on the Varishaker (speed 3–4, about 600–1000 rpm). The enzymic reaction was then stopped by the addition of 50 µl of 2.5 M sulphuric acid to each well.

The Magnogel complex was separated from the liquid phase (i.e. chromogenic product) by use of the magnet and a sample (50 µl) of the liquid phase was transferred to corresponding wells in a microtitre plate containing 150 µl of distilled water. The absorbance of diluted product was then measured at 490 nm using a Micro ELISA reader (Model MR590; Dynatech Laboratories).

Standard Curve for Enterotoxin B using MEIA

Typical standard curves for enterotoxin B are shown in Fig. 2. These results are from duplicate tests done on a single occasion. The lower limit of sensitivity of the

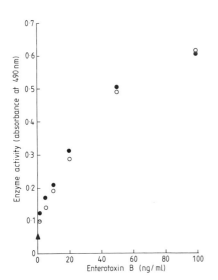
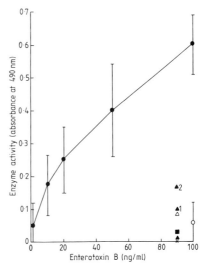

FIG. 2. Titration of standard staphylococcal enterotoxin B against a constant level of anti-enterotoxin B-coupled Magnogel. ●, ○, duplicate samples on one occasion; ▲, control (antibody-coupled Magnogel, no enterotoxin B).

FIG. 3. Titration of standard enterotoxin B against a constant level of anti-enterotoxin B-coupled Magnogel. Ι, standard deviation; ○, control, no enterotoxin, n = 13; ●, standard enterotoxin B, n = 20; x, enterotoxin A (0.1–3 µg/ml); △, enterotoxin C (0.1–10 µg/ml); ■, enterotoxin D (0.1–10 µg/ml); enterotoxin E, ▲ 0.1 µg/ml; ▲₁, 1 µg/ml; ▲₂, 10 µg/ml.

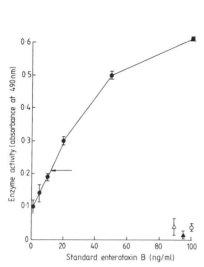

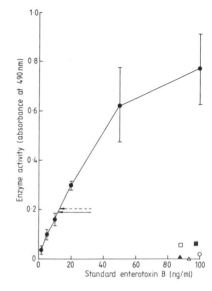

FIG. 4. Estimation of enterotoxin B in cheese by the direct MEIA technique. Ɪ, standard deviation of 4 points; ●, standard enterotoxin B; ○, control (no enterotoxin); △, cheese extract (no enterotoxin); ▲, cheese extract with enterotoxin E; ← cheese extract with enterotoxin B.

FIG. 5. Estimation of enterotoxin B in ham and chicken-liver pâté by the direct MEIA technique. Ɪ, standard deviation of 4 points; ●, standard enterotoxin B; ○, control (no enterotoxin); △, □, ham extract; ▲, ■, chicken-liver pâté extract; △, ▲, no enterotoxin B; □, ■, enterotoxin E (1 μg/100 g); ←ham extract, ←--chicken-liver pâté extract, with enterotoxin B.

assay is 10 ng/ml. Results from replicate assays done on different days show more variability (Fig. 3); therefore it is necessary to perform an assay for a set of standard enterotoxin B concentrations on each occasion. The MEIA showed specificity for enterotoxin B except for a slight cross-reaction with enterotoxin E at high concentration (Fig. 3).

Estimation of Enterotoxin B Extracted from Foods

The recovery of staphylococcal enterotoxin B added to foods, estimated by MEIA, is shown in Table 1. Recovery was variable for all the foods, which means that the estimation of enterotoxin B can be at best only semi-quantitative. Estimations, by the MEIA technique, of pure enterotoxin B added to foods (1 μg/100 g) are shown for Cheddar cheese (Fig. 4), ham and chicken liver pâté (Fig. 5) and skimmed milk powder (Fig. 6). A result could be obtained in 6–7 h.

TABLE 1.   *Recovery of enterotoxin B from various foods*

Food	Estimation of % recovery in food extract	
	Mean	Range
Cheese	110	93–120
Skimmed milk powder	80	40–106
Ham	70	60–80
Chicken liver pâté	130	113–146

Estimation of Enterotoxin B Produced by *Staph. aureus* in Ham

The amount of enterotoxin produced by *Staph. aureus* NCTC 10654 grown in ham was about 11.5 µg enterotoxin B/100 g ham as estimated by the direct MEIA (Fig. 7). In contrast, low enzyme activity was exhibited in the MEIA technique by the extracts of ham inoculated with non-enterotoxigenic *Staph. aureus* NCTC 7121 (equivalent to 100 ng enterotoxin B/100 g ham) and *Staph. aureus* NCTC 8530 (equivalent to 600 ng enterotoxin B/100 g ham).

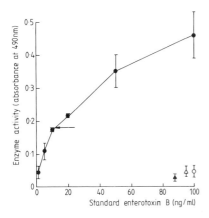

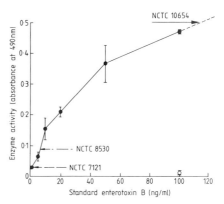

FIG. 6.   Estimation of enterotoxin B in dried skimmed milk by the direct MEIA technique. $\mathbf{I}$, standard deviation of 4 points; ●, standard enterotoxin B; ○, control (no enterotoxin); △, milk extract, no enterotoxin; ▲, milk extract, enterotoxin E (1 µg/100 g); ←milk extract with enterotoxin B.

FIG. 7.   Estimation of enterotoxin B produced in ham by *Staph. aureus*. $\mathbf{I}$, standard deviation of 4 points; ●, standard enterotoxin B; ○, no enterotoxin B. Arrows represent readings from ham extracts containing *Staph. aureus* strains.

Effect of protein A on the direct MEIA technique

The interference by protein A ($\geqslant 10$ ng/ml) in the direct MEIA is shown in Fig. 8. High levels of protein A ($\geqslant 10$ ng/100 g food) are required to cause interference. Data in Fig. 7 demonstrate that the extract of ham contaminated with *Staph. aureus* NCTC 8530 (a known protein A producer) caused more interference with the MEIA technique than did *Staph. aureus* NCTC 7121. This result suggests that > 50 ng protein A/100 g ham (from Fig. 8) is produced by this strain of *Staph. aureus* (NCTC 8530) and may cause false positive results for enterotoxin although at a very low level.

The interference by protein A with enterotoxin estimation in extracts of cheese is shown in Fig. 9. Approximately 100% of enterotoxin B was recovered from the cheese extract in the absence of protein A. In the presence of protein A, however,

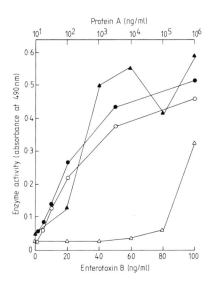

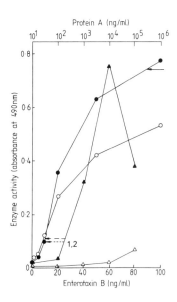

FIG. 8. Inteference by protein A in the direct MEIA technique. ●, standard enterotoxin B; ○, standard enterotoxin B+Spicer–Edwards antiserum; ▲, protein A; △, protein A+ Spicer-Edwards antiserum. All points represent the mean of four replicates.

FIG. 9. Estimation of enterotoxin B in cheese, in the presence of protein A, by the direct MEIA technique. Legends as FIG. 8, plus ←cheese extract+enterotoxin B+protein A (1 mg/ 100 g); ←———cheese extract+enterotoxin B; 1 ←------cheese extract+enterotoxin B+ protein A (1 mg/100 g)+Spicer–Edwards antiserum; 2 ←------cheese extract+enterotoxin B+Spicer–Edwards antiserum.

the recovery of enterotoxin B was apparently about 900%. The interference by protein A for concentrations up to 10 μg/ml was eliminated by reacting the protein A-containing solution with non-enterotoxin-specific rabbit antibodies (pooled Spicer–Edwards *Salmonella* H antiserum) prior to the MEIA technique (Figs. 8 and 9).

Conclusions

An MEIA has been developed which allows the detection of $\leqslant 1$ μg enterotoxin B/100 g food within a working day. This is considerably faster than the conventional technique (which takes at least a week) and also quicker than currently available kits, which require 24–30 h to obtain a result. Work is currently progressing to extend the technique to the other staphylococcal enterotoxins.

The MEIA is simple to operate as separation and washing procedures are easily achieved by use of a magnet. The major practical problem with the MEIA technique is that it is difficult to dispense equal quantities of the Magnogel between occasions, as shown by the variability in Fig. 4, as opposed to within occasions (Fig. 3). A standard curve must therefore be prepared on each occasion.

Interference by protein A in the assay can be virtually eliminated by using non-enterotoxin-specific antibodies, thus preventing false-positive results due to the presence of protein A-producing *Staph. aureus*. The technique will probably be of use as a semi-quantitative test, rather than a fully quantitative test, due to the variation in recoveries of enterotoxin achieved between occasions.

Appendix I

Purification of anti-enterotoxin IgG antibodies by affinity chromatography using protein A Sepharose CL-4B gel

Preparation of anti-enterotoxin serum

Freeze-dried antiserum B (200 mg/ml; gift from Professor J. Melling) was reconstituted in 1 ml of 0.1 M phosphate buffer, pH 7.0, and desalted using PD-10 columns of Sephadex G-25M (Pharmacia Fine Chemicals, UK) according to the manufacturer's instructions. Desalted protein solution (about 2 ml) was concentrated to about 0.7 ml by dialysis against 40% w/v polyethylene glycol (mol.wt. 20 000; Sigma) at 4 °C for about 4 h. If the solution was cloudy, it was centrifuged (2000 g for 5 min) and the clear supernatant (0.65 ml) was applied to a column of protein A Sepharose CL4B.

Protein A Sepharose CL-4B gel

Protein A, isolated from the Cowan 1 strain of *Staph. aureus*, binds specifically with IgG-type antibodies. It interacts with the F_c portion of IgG molecules, thus leaving two F_{ab} portions for normal immunological reactions. Protein A Sepharose CL-4B (Sigma) is the gel Sepharose CL-4B to which protein A has been covalently coupled by the cyanogen bromide method.

Preparation of protein A Sepharose CL-4B column

Protein A Sepharose CL-4B (500 mg) was reconstituted in 15 ml of 0.1 M phosphate buffer, pH 7.0, and allowed to swell for 15 min. An empty PD-10 column (1.5 cm diameter; Pharmacia Fine Chemicals) was mounted vertically and the lower end was connected via silicone tubing to a peristaltic pump (Varioperpex; LKB Ltd), a Uvicord S (model 2138; LKB Ltd) and a fraction collector (model 7000; LKB Ltd). The absorbance at 280 nm monitored by the Uvicord S was recorded on a chart recorder (model 2210; LKB Ltd). The swollen gel was deaerated under vacuum and guided into the PD-10 column by a glass rod. When a thin layer of gel had settled, the packing flow rate was adjusted to about 0.5 ml/min with the pump. The settled gel (bed dimensions 1.5 cm diameter × 11 cm height) was then washed and equilibrated with about 500 ml deaerated 0.1 M phosphate buffer, pH 7.0, at a flow rate of 0.4 ml/min.

Application of antiserum and chromatographic elution

Antiserum (1 ml) was applied to the column with a Pasteur pipette and drained into the bed at a flow rate of about 0.4 ml/min. The pump was stopped and the column was filled with 1 ml of 0.1 M phosphate buffer, pH 7.0, in order to prevent the bed from drying. The column was allowed to stand at ambient temperature for 30 min to allow the pseudo-immune reaction between protein A and antibodies to occur.

The equilibration buffer was placed in a buffer reservoir (LKB 2137–036; LKB Ltd), which was then connected via the polyethylene tube to the upper end of the column. The column was then eluted with the equilibration buffer at a flow rate of 1 ml/min. The effluent was monitored at 280 nm and 2 ml fractions were collected.

The first peak from the column comprised excess proteins, including unbound immunoglobulins. The second peak was eluted with 0.1 M glycine-HCl (0.2 M) buffer, pH 3.0. The fractions comprising the peak were pooled (about 10 ml) and dialysed against 1 litre of 0.1 M phosphate buffer, pH 7.0 (at 4 °C for 16 h) and the volume in the dialysis sac (about 10 ml) was then reduced to about 0.5 ml by further dialysis against 20% w/v polyethylene glycol (at 4 °C for 4 h). The concentrated IgG solution was tested for immunological activity by double immunodiffusion. The purified IgG was used for coupling to peroxidase.

Appendix II

Coupling of peroxidase to staphylococcal enterotoxin B purified IgG antibodies

The procedure was followed as described in the instruction manual for 'N-succinimidyl 3-(2-pyridyldithio) propionate (SPDP) Heterobifunctional reagent' supplied by Pharmacia Fine Chemicals (1978). The following stages were involved in this procedure.

Purified IgG preparation (0.5 ml) was dialysed against 1 litre of 0.1 M phosphate buffer (pH 7.5, containing 0.1 M sodium chloride) at 4 °C for 24 h. The dialysed IgG was then made up to 1 ml in the same buffer.

Horseradish peroxidase (8 mg) was dissolved in 1 ml 0.1 M phosphate buffer (pH 7.5, containing 0.1 M sodium chloride) and SPDP was dissolved in absolute ethanol to a concentration of 40 mM. A portion (25 μl) of the SPDP was quickly added to the IgG and horseradish peroxidase preparations and allowed to react for 30 min at ambient temperature (about 20 °C). This procedure added 2-pyridyl residues to the proteins from SPDP.

The SPDP-coupled IgG solution was then dialysed (16 h at 4 °C) against 1 litre of 0.1 M phosphate buffer, pH 7.5, containing 0.1 M sodium chloride. The SPDP-coupled peroxidase solution was dialysed against 1 litre of 0.1 M sodium acetate buffer, pH 4.5, containing 0.1 M sodium chloride for 16 h at 4 °C. Dithiothreitol (a reducing agent) was then added to the dialysed protein to a final concentration of 50 mM and mixed for 20 min at ambient temperature. Excess dithiothreitol and pyridine-2-thione (a by-product of the reaction) were removed by passing the protein solution through a PD-10 Sephadex column (Pharmacia Fine Chemicals) previously equilibrated with 0.1 M phosphate buffer, pH 7.5, containing 0.1 M sodium chloride. The dithiothreitol treatment reduces the 2-pyridyl disulphide groups of the peroxidase.

The SPDP-peroxidase and SPDP-IgG solutions were then mixed and allowed to react for 24 h at ambient temperature using a magnetic stirrer, to form the antibody-enzyme conjugate. The conjugate solution (about 4.5 ml) was dialysed against 1 litre of 30% w/v polyethylene glycol for 18 h at 4 °C to reduce the volume to approximately 1.5 ml and then dialysed further against 1 litre of 0.1 M phosphate buffer, pH 7.5, containing 0.1 M sodium chloride, at 4 °C for 18 h. High molecular weight conjugates were separated from the reactants by gel permeation chromatography.

References

BERGDOLL, M. S. & REISER, R. F. 1980 Application of radioimmunoassay for detection of staphylococcal enterotoxins in foods. *Journal of Food Protection* **43**, 68–72.

BOOTHROYD, M. & BAIRD-PARKER, A. C. 1973 The use of enrichment serology for *Salmonella* detection in human foods and animal feeds. *Journal of Applied Bacteriology* **36**, 165–172.

CROWLE, A. J. 1958 A simplified micro double-diffusion agar precipitin technique. *Journal of Laboratory and Clinical Medicine* **52**, 784.

GUESDON, J. L. & AVRAMEAS, S. 1977 Magnetic solid phase enzyme-immunoassay. *Immunochemistry* **14**, 443–447.

HOLBROOK, R. & BAIRD-PARKER, A. C. 1975 Serological methods for the assay of staphylococcal enterotoxins. In *Some Methods for Microbiological Analysis* SAB Technical Series No. 8, eds. Board, R. G. & Lovelock, D. W. pp. 107–126. London: Academic Press.

NISKANEN, A. 1977 *Staphylococcal Enterotoxins and Food Poisoning.* Publication No. 19, Technical Research Centre of Finland.

NOTERMANS, S., BOOT, R., TIPS, P. D. & NOOIJ, M. P. DE. 1983 Extraction of staphylococcal enterotoxins (SE) from minced meat and subsequent detection of SE with enzyme-linked immunosorbent assay (ELISA). *Journal of Food Protection* **46**, 238–241.

VOLLER, A., BIDWELL, D. E. & BARTLETT, A. 1979 *The Enzyme Linked Immunosorbent Assay (ELISA).* Available from: Dynatech Europe, Guernsey, Channel Islands, U.K.

WOOD, J. M. & PAYNE, D. N. 1974 Convenient micro system for double diffusion immunoprecipitin tests. *Laboratory Practice* **Dec.** 695–698.

The Potential Use of Monoclonal Antibodies in the Diagnosis of Tuberculosis

P. S. Jackett

MRC Tuberculosis and Related Infections Unit, Hammersmith Hospital, Ducane Road, London W12 0HS

Introduction

The successful treatment of tuberculosis, once diagnosed, depends upon effective therapeutic regimens and drug compliance. The current repertoire of antituberculosis drugs provides many good regimens for treatment, but poorer countries find the better drug combinations prohibitively expensive. However, the control and eventual elimination of tuberculosis depends upon both effective therapy and the prevention of transmission of infection prior to diagnosis and treatment. Indeed, both socio-economically and epidemiologically, prevention is better than cure. Reduction in the spread of tuberculosis would undoubtedly be achieved by improvements in housing and hygiene, by diagnosis of disease prior to sputum positivity and by the development of better vaccines.

Diagnosis of pulmonary tuberculosis is based upon a combination of criteria including symptoms, tuberculin skin test, chest radiograph and sputum smear and culture. In many Third World countries there is great dependence upon the direct smear examination, which only becomes positive for acid-fast bacilli when the disease is advanced and the patient has already transmitted bacilli and infected susceptible contacts. Even where good culture facilities are available, which can identify the smear-negative, culture-positive patients, their value is diminished by the delay of up to 8 weeks awaiting the result, during which time the risk of further cross-infection is ever increasing. Thus new methods of early diagnosis of tuberculosis are needed. Recognition of this need has inspired the search for a serological test for tuberculosis for over 80 years.

Titres of antibodies against the different antigenic determinants of the infecting organism are raised during the course of bacterial disease. Although resistance to tuberculosis is a result of cell-mediated immunity rather than a humoral response, antibodies are nevertheless produced against *Mycobacterium tuberculosis* antigens following infection. However the specificity of these antibodies ranges from the

Immunological Techniques
in Microbiology

species-specific, to those which cross-react with antigenic determinants common to other mycobacteria and even unrelated organisms. The comparative failure of previous serological tests for tuberculosis has been due both to the overlap between healthy controls and patients due to these cross-reactive epitopes, together with the lack of antibody response in some patients, possibly due to individual variations in the immune response.

The advent and application of monoclonal antibodies (MAbs) to specific antigenic epitopes has provided the potential to improve the specificity of immunoassays on sera and other body fluids. Serologically, they have, to date, been exploited in two ways. First, their specificity of epitope binding has been used to develop a solid-phase antibody competition test (SACT) which does not require pre-purification of antigens. The test using MAbs derived from murine Balb/c-NS1 hybridomas, has been applied to tuberculosis (Coates *et al.*, 1981; Hewitt *et al.*, 1982; Ivanyi *et al.*, 1983; Hoeppner *et al.*, 1987) and leprosy (Sinha *et al.*, 1983, 1985). Secondly, the technique of column-affinity chromatography has enabled mycobacterial antigens to be purified from crude culture filtrates or extracts (Ivanyi *et al.*, 1985; Young *et al.*, 1986). The use of the pure antigens should provide the basis for a serological assay of greater specificity than those previously described (Grange, 1984). The techniques and current status of these two potential applications are discussed in this chapter.

Where antibody detection may not be possible, detection of mycobacterial antigen has been reported as a possible alternative. A 'Tandem' immunoassay has been developed using one MAb (ML34) which is specific for a protease-resistant cell-wall constituent lipoarabinomannan B (LAM-B) (Praputpittaya & Ivanyi, 1985; Hunter *et al.*, 1986). Since the binding site on the antigenic molecule is a

TABLE 1. *The monoclonal antibodies used in the assays described in this chapter, with their specificities of binding to mycobacterial antigens*

Monoclonal antibody		Antigen		Binding specificity		
code	Ig	molecular weight (× 1000)	structure	*M. tuberculosis* complex	*M. leprae*	other mycobacteria
TB68	G1	11–14	Protein	+	−	—
TB23	G1	19	Protein	+	−	limited
TB71	G2b	38	Protein	+*	−	—
TB72	G1			+	−	—
TB78	G1	65	Protein	+	−	limited
ML34	M	25–40	Saccharide	+	+	broad

*TB71 and TB72 bind to two distinct epitopes on the 38 000 molecule.

repeating sequence, the antibody can be used as both the solid-phase capture reagent and the labelled second antibody. The principle of the assay has also been applied previously where separate MAbs are available to two distinct epitopes on protein antigens which do not carry repeating determinants (Sevier *et al.*, 1981; Uotila *et al.*, 1981; Soos & Siddle, 1982). This variation has been used with the MAbs TB71 and TB72 which bind to distinct epitopes of the 38 kd soluble protein antigen which is specific to *M. tuberculosis* (Young *et al.*, 1986). This technique is described here, together with a further application of the ML34 antibody for antigen detection by reverse passive haemagglutination (Chandramuki *et al.*, 1985). The monoclonal antibodies used in the assays described in this chapter, with their specificities of binding to mycobacterial antigens, are shown in Table 1.

Methods

The solid-phase antibody competition assay (SACT)

The principle of the SACT assay is shown in Fig. 1a. A soluble extract of *M. tuberculosis*, strain H37Rv, (MTSE) at a predetermined optimal concentration, is coated onto a solid-phase. The serum is then allowed to compete for binding to the coated antigens with the radiolabelled (as illustrated) or enzyme-conjugated monoclonal antibody.

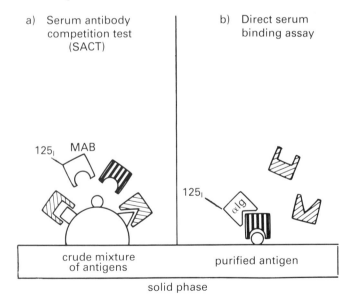

FIG. 1. Schematic representation of a) the serum antibody competition test; b) the direct serum binding assay.

Iodination of monoclonal antibodies (MAbs)

MAbs are iodinated by the iodogen technique (Fraker & Speck, 1978) and separated from free iodine by ion exchange chromatography.

PRELIMINARY PROCEDURE

Column preparation: the columns are prepared by making a paste of Dowex-1 (Sigma Chemical Co.) with 1% bovine serum albumin (BSA) in phosphate-buffered saline (Dulbecco A, PBS) containing 0.1% (w/v) solium azide (NaN_3) and filling a 2 ml plastic disposable syringe (without plunger) fitted with a dropper. Small discs of Whatman GF/B filters are fitted at the bottom and top of the column. The column is washed and stabilized with 1% BSA.

Sample: 50 µg of MAb is pipetted in a volume of 100 µl into a microfuge tube (1.2 ml capacity).

PROCEDURE IN 'HOT-LAB'

The MAb is transferred into an iodogen-coated microfuge tube. After mixing, the tube is placed in the fume-cupboard and 0.5 mCi of Na ^{125}I is added (approximately 5 µl). The tube is incubated for 12 min with gentle tapping each min. Two hundred microlitres of PBS is then added to the tube and the total volume (approximately 300 µl) is transferred to the column. The resulting eluent is discarded. After standing for 1 min, the column is then washed with 4×0.5 ml aliquots of 1% BSA and the total 2 ml eluent containing the iodinated antibody is collected in a plastic Bijou bottle (containing a few crystals of NaN_3) and placed in a lead container. Estimates are then made of the total radioactivity recovered and the percentage of that amount which is protein-bound. This should be $> 90\%$. The estimate is done by co-precipitation with 1% BSA by trichloracetic acid (TCA). Briefly, 5 µl of radiolabelled antibody is mixed with 0.5 ml of 1% BSA and 0.5 ml of 20% (w/v) TCA, incubated for more than 3 h at 4 °C and then centrifuged at 1000 g for 10 min. The supernatant is discarded and the precipitate counted, in parallel with an untreated 5 µl sample, in the gamma counter.

Peroxidase-conjugation of MAbs

The production of peroxidase-conjugated MAbs was generously undertaken by Dr Julian Duncan at Wellcome Laboratories, Beckenham.

Preparation of MTSE

M. tuberculosis, strain $H_{37}Rv$, is grown for 8 weeks as a surface pellicle on Sauton's medium. The bacilli are then separated from the growth medium by centrifugation at 3000 g. The medium, which is also rich in antigens, is then rendered safe for use by filtration (Millipore or Durapore, 0.45 μm). The bacilli are irradiated (2.5 megarad, ^{59}Co) before disruption.

DISRUPTION PROCESS USING A BRAUN HOMOGENISER

Ten gram bacilli, wet weight, are suspended in 10 ml cold PBS. The ice-cold suspension is placed in a pre-cooled homogeniser bottle, which already contains 50 g glass beads, diameter 0.1–0.11 mm. Two hundred microlitres of 200 μM phenyl methyl sulphonyl fluoride (PMSF) in ethanol are added. The homogeniser chamber is pre-cooled by passing a stream of CO_2 through it and the stream is left running during disruption. The machine is operated at 4000 rpm for 2 min during which time the sample should remain cool, but not frozen. The homogenate is separated from the beads by allowing it to settle for 2–3 min and then removing it by pipette. The pooled homogenate is then centrifuged at 47 000 g for 1 h at 4 °C. The pooled supernatant is aliquoted and stored at -20 °C. A small aliquot is retained for protein estimation and testing (see next paragraph). Ten grams of *M. tuberculosis* will usually yield more than 30 mg of protein, sufficient for 200 radioimmunoassay (RIA) plates or 600 ELISA plates.

Testing of MTSE

The MTSE is diluted to 100 μg/ml protein in PBS. Microtitre plates are coated (50 μl/well) with concentrations of MTSE at 100, 30, 10, 3, 1 and 0 μg/ml diluted in PBS, for the following assay:

1 For RIA, using flexible 96 well plates with U-shaped wells (Dynatech). Plates are coated overnight at 4 °C at 50 μl/well then washed once with PBS (note: for all assays, all incubations are carried out in a humidified container). The wells are blocked with 200 μl of 3% BSA (in PBS) for 1 h at room temperature, then washed twice with PBS. The unlabelled MAbs are then added (50 μl/well) at a dilution of 4 μg/ml in 3% BSA (TB23, 68, 71, 72, 78 and ML34) and incubated for 4 h at room temperature. After washing three times with PBS, 30 000 cpm/well of ^{125}I-labelled rabbit anti-mouse Ig $F(ab)_2$ in 50 μl of 3% BSA are added and incubated overnight at 4 °C. The plates are then washed five times with PBS, cut up and counted in the gamma counter.

2 For ELISA, using rigid plates (Dynatech Immulon M129B). Plates are coated overnight at 4 °C, then washed once with PBS containing 0.05% (v/v) Tween 20 (PBS-Tween). The wells are blocked with 200 μl PBS-Tween for 1 h at 37 °C, after

which the PBS-Tween is tipped off and the plates patted dry. The MAbs are added as for the RIA, but diluted in PBS-Tween. The subsequent incubation is for 1 h at 37 °C. After washing three times with PBS-Tween, 50 µl/well of an affinity purified anti-mouse Ig-horseradish peroxidase conjugate, diluted in PBS-Tween to the recommended or evaluated concentration (usually 1/1000 or 1/3000) are added and the plates incubated for a further 1 h at 37 °C. The plates are then washed three times with PBS-Tween, and patted dry for the addition of substrate.

Preparation of substrate for ELISA-peroxidase-conjugate assays

The recommended substrate is tetramethyl benzidine in combination with hydrogen peroxide in citrate buffer pH 5.1 (TMB/H_2O_2). It is prepared by dissolving the required amount of TMB in a small quantity of water, then transferring the solution to the correct volume of buffer to a final concentration of 0.1 mg/ml. The H_2O_2 is added immediately before the reaction by a 1–4 in 10 000 dilution of a 30% (w/v) stock solution of H_2O_2 (i.e. 0.1–0.4 µl/ml). It is important not to add excess H_2O_2, or substrate inhibition will occur. The reaction is started by the addition of 75 µl substrate to each well. The reaction is stopped after 10 min at room temperature by the addition of 50 µl/well of 0.5 M H_2SO_4, which also changes the developed blue colour to yellow. The absorbance is subsequently read in a Titertek Multiskan Spectrophotometer (Flow Laboratories) at 450 nm.

For each of the assays described the optimal coating concentration of MTSE is the lowest at which all six MAbs give saturating coating (i.e. maximal cpm or optical density respectively).

The SACT assay: RIA

Antigen coating: MTSE is coated by the addition of 50 µl/well of the predetermined optimal dilution in PBS (usually 30 µg/ml) onto 96 well plates (Dynatech flexible, U-shaped). Incubation is overnight at 4 °C, followed by one wash with PBS. For each antibody two wells are left uncoated for low controls.

Blocking: the wells are filled with 3% BSA in PBS and incubated for 1 h at room temperature, followed by two washes with PBS.

Sample addition: chosen dilutions of test sera are added (25 µl) and incubated for 4 h at room temperature. Usual dilutions are 1/5, 1/25, 1/125 and 1/625 in 3% BSA. Low controls and high controls contain only 3% BSA.

Competition: 25 µl of ^{125}I-MAb diluted in 3% BSA are added at 30 000 cpm/well or at appropriate dilutions to give a high control of 1000–2000 cpm/well. Incubation is overnight at 4 °C after thorough mixing. 2 × 25 µl aliquots are retained to estimate the counts added. After five washes with PBS, plates are dried (30–60 min, room temperature) and counted.

Low control: (no coating antigen) binding of ^{125}I-MAb to BSA-blocked wells.

High control: (no competition) binding of ^{125}I-MAb alone to antigen.

The SACT assay: ELISA

Antigen coating: Dynatech Immulon (M129B) plates are coated with 50 µl/well of MTSE (usually 10 µg/ml) diluted in PBS (PBS only for low controls). Incubation is overnight at 4 °C, followed by one wash with PBS-Tween.

Blocking: the wells are filled with PBS-Tween (150–200 µl) and incubated for 1 h at 37 °C. Then the PBS-Tween is tipped off and the plates patted dry.

Sample addition: chosen dilutions of sera (25 µl/well) or 25 µl PBS-Tween for high and low controls are added and the plates incubated for 1 h at 37 °C.

Competition: 25 µl/well of MAb-peroxidase conjugate are added at that dilution (in PBS-Tween) which will give 90% maximal binding in the absence of competition (high control). Incubation is for 2 h at 37 °C. After four washes with PBS-Tween, the plates are shaken as dry as possible and wiped clean on the underside. The substrate (TMB/H_2O_2) is added and the reaction stopped (H_2SO_4) as described earlier.

Low control: (no coating antigen) binding of conjugate to PBS-Tween-blocked wells only.

High Control: (no serum) binding of conjugate to antigen without competition.

Calculation of results

The results are expressed as the antibody titre which will inhibit binding of the iodinated, or conjugated, MAb to the solid-phase-bound antigens by 50% and is called the ABT_{50}. Mathematically, it is the inverse of the dilution that gives 50% inhibition and that value may, and probably will, differ from antibody to antibody. An example is given in Fig. 2. In practice, the result is calculated by intrapolation from the straight line between the two serum dilutions which are either side of the 50% inhibition value.

Application of the RIA-SACT assay

The first small study in Britain using MAbs TB23, TB68 and TB72 resulted in no positives in sera from 30 healthy controls, and 71% positives amongst 41 smear-

　　　　　　　　　　P. S. JACKETT

Serum antibody titration

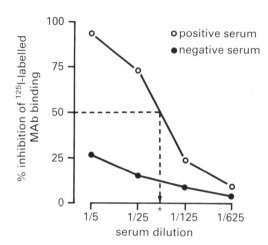

FIG. 2.　Titration curves of typical positive and negative sera to establish the competing serum antibody titre. *The 50% inhibition titres are calculated for each Mab for each serum.

positive tuberculosis patients (Hewitt *et al.*, 1982). A more recent study (Hoeppner *et al.*, 1987), on 34 healthy Indonesian controls and 100 smear-positive patients, yielded a positivity amongst patients of >90% with no positives in the controls. Sinha *et al.* (1985) assayed sera from leprosy patients and controls, for antibodies which competed with the MAb ML04 for binding to soluble protein extract of *Mycobacterium leprae*. They achieved positive results with 100% sera from lepromatous and borderline lepromatous (LL and BL) patients (Ridley & Jopling, 1966), seven out of eight from borderline (BB) patients, 50% from LL, BL and BB contacts, and tuberculoid and borderline tuberculoid (TT and BT) patients, but with no sera from healthy subjects and other control groups.

Direct binding assay

Principle of assay: the principle of this assay is shown in Fig. 1b. Purified antigen from *M. tuberculosis* extract, or culture filtrate, is coated onto Immulon plates and the binding of serum antibodies to the antigen is detected with peroxidase-conjugated second antibody.

Purification of antigens

Antigens are purified by immunoaffinity chromatography, using the MAbs already described. The method of purification is as described by Young *et al.* (1986). The globulin fraction, precipitated by 18% Na_2SO_4, from ascitic fluid of one of the MAbs is coupled to cyanogen-bromide-activated Sepharose 4B according to the manufacturer's (Pharmacia) instructions, using 7.5 mg protein/ml of gel. The column (6 ml) is prepared for use by washing with PBS and elution buffers and stored in PBS with 0.1% sodium azide. The culture filtrate or extract is passed down the column at a flow rate of approximately 30 ml/h and the columns are washed with PBS until no further protein is eluted. The bound material is then eluted with four column volumes each of a succession of three buffers which are: (1) 1.0 M NaCl; (2) 0.1 M glycine/HCl pH 2.5; and (3) 10% (v/v) dioxan in 0.1 M glycine/HCl, pH 2.5. The column can be re-equilibrated with PBS and stored for further use. Five millilitre fractions are collected during elution and assayed for antigenic binding activity by ELISA and protein concentrations are estimated by using BSA as a standard.

Testing of antigen coating

The optimal coating concentrations of purified 19 kd and 38 kd antigens which discriminate maximally between positive and negative sera are estimated by coating serial dilutions of the antigen in PBS onto Immulon plates and measuring the binding to sera of known high competitive inhibitory titres to TB23 and TB71/72 respectively (previously determined by SACT) with peroxidase–conjugated second antibody (affinity-purified goat anti-human IgG (gamma chain) (Sigma)).

Method of direct antigen binding assay

Antigen coating: immulon plates are coated with 50 µl/well of antigen (19 kd, 38 kd or PBS for control of non specific binding of each serum) and incubated overnight at 4 °C followed by one wash with PBS-Tween.

Blocking: the wells are blocked with PBS-Tween (200 µl) by incubating for 1 h at 37 °C. The PBS-Tween is tipped out and shaken off as much as possible.

Sample addition: fifty microlitres of the appropriate dilutions of test or control sera, diluted in PBS-Tween are added to the wells and the plates incubated for 1 h at 37 °C. A positive standard (high control, 2 wells/plate) is added to calculate 100% binding.

Second antibody: following three washes with PBS-Tween, 50 µl of goat anti-human IgG peroxidase conjugate (γ chain specific, affinity purified, Sigma) diluted in PBS-Tween (1/1000) are added and the plates are incubated for a further 1 h at 37 °C. The plates are washed three times with PBS-Tween. All excess wash is shaken off and the plates are wiped clean for reaction with TMB/H_2O_2 substrate as described earlier.

Calculations

The percentage binding of each serum at each test dilution is calculated relative to the high control after allowance for non-specific binding in the absence of antigen. The cut-off percentage binding value to enable optimal discrimination between control and tuberculosis patients' sera must be evaluated for each antigen. Preliminary investigations have shown promise for both antigens. Sera from eight patients with active pulmonary tuberculosis were compared with seven control sera for binding to 19 kd-coated plates. Estimates of the serum titres which gave 25% binding yielded values of < 1 to 58 for the controls, and 86 to > 625 for the patients. A similar pattern of results was obtained for the 38 kd-binding assay (Young *et al.*, 1986).

Antigen capture assays

The 'tandem' or sandwich assay for the detection of the LAM-B antigen (previously known as MY-4) common to *M. tuberculosis* and *M. leprae* extracts was first described by Praputpittaya & Ivanyi (1985) and applied by Chandramuki *et al.* (1985) to cerebrospinal fluid (CSF). The principle of the method demands either an antigen with repeating epitopes for a single MAb (as with LAM-B and ML34) or an antigen with two distinct epitopes (at least) and the two complementary MAbs (as with the 38 kd protein and TB71 and TB72). Thus, in the ML34 assay, the MAb, which binds to the polysaccharide antigen, is used both on the solid phase as the coating antibody and as the ^{125}I-labelled or peroxidase-conjugated tracer antibody. The detection of the 38 kd antigen is done by coating with TB71, adding the samples containing antigen and tracing with ^{125}I-labelled TB72. Interestingly, the reverse procedure (TB72 followed by ^{125}I-TB71) works less well.

Method of ML34 'tandem' antigen capture assay: RIA

Dynatech 96 well plates (flexible, U-shaped wells) are coated with ML34 (50 μl/ well) at 10 μg/ml in PBS and incubated overnight at 4 °C. After one wash with PBS the wells are blocked with 3% BSA for 1 h at room temperature. The plates are then washed twice with PBS before sample addition. CSF samples are used undiluted and at 1 in 2, 1 in 4 and 1 in 8 dilutions at 50 μl/well. Standards are included of MTSE at 32 μg/ml and at seven further twofold dilutions (to 250 ng/ml), or of eight similar dilutions of purified LAM-B ranging from 4 μg/ml to 31.25 ng/ml. The incubation is for 2 h at 37 °C, followed by three washes with PBS. ^{125}I-labelled ML34 is then added at 30 000 cpm/well and the plates incubated for a further 2 h at 37 °C. The plates are then washed five times, dried and counted.

Method of ML34 'tandem' antigen capture assay: ELISA

Rigid Immulon plates are coated with 10 μg/ml ML34 (50 μl/well). After incubation at 4 °C, overnight, the plates are washed once then blocked with PBS-Tween for

1 h at 37 °C. The PBS-Tween is tipped off and the samples and standards diluted in PBS-Tween are added at 50 µl/well. After incubation for 1 h at 37 °C the plates are washed twice with PBS-Tween and peroxidase-conjugated ML34 added at 50 µl/well. The dilution of ML34 is determined for each batch, but is usually 1 in 2000, or 1 in 4000. The final incubation is for 2 h at 37 °C. After three washes with PBS-Tween, the TMB/H_2O_2 substrate is added as described earlier.

Detection of 38 kd antigen—RIA

The incubation conditions are as described for the ML34 'tandem' assay with the following substitutions; coating is done with TB71 at 5 µg/ml; the range of standards using MTSE is the same as for LAM-B detection with ML34, but 38 kd standards are also included at 500 ng/ml and at seven further twofold dilutions; ^{125}I-labelled TB72 is added at 90 000 cpm/well.

Detection of LAM-B antigen by reverse passive haemagglutination

This is an alternative method of detecting the LAM-B antigenic component of mycobacteria, using the ML34 antibody as described by Chandramuki et al. (1985). Chymotrypsin-treated sheep red blood cells (SRBC) are coupled to the IgM MAb ML34, which had been prepared by precipitation from ascitic fluid with 18% sodium sulphate. Haemagglutination occurs on interaction with the multivalent LAM-B molecule.

Chymotrypsin-treatment of SRBC: the SRBC are washed five times by centrifugation in PBS at 4 °C for 5 min at 300 g at a proportion of 10 vol of PBS to 1 vol of packed cells. The cells are resuspended in the same proportion. Chymotrypsin solution (bovine pancreas, type II, Sigma) is prepared at 5 mg/ml in 1 mM HCl/0.9% NaCl and warmed to 37 °C. One volume is mixed with 4 vol of prewarmed complement fixation test diluent buffer (CFT, Oxoid). The mixture is added to 5 vol of prewarmed SRBC. After 20 min incubation at 37 °C the cells are washed twice with PBS at room temperature for 5 min at 1000 g. The pellet is then resuspended in an equal volume of a 1 in 40 dilution of trypsin inhibitor (soybean, Sigma) and incubated at room temperature for 10 min. Physiological saline (0.9% NaCl) is added and the cells are washed three times by centrifugation at 1000 g for 10 min. The supernatant is decanted carefully and the cells are kept at 4 °C for use.

Coupling procedure: the method is that described by Scott et al. (1981), using chromic chloride. The optimal concentrations of ML34 and chromic chloride are established by chequerboard titration over the ranges 100 to 1000 µg/ml and 1 in 30 to 1 in 45 dilutions of a 1% solution in 0.9% NaCl respectively. Typically, 50 µl of a 1 in 30 dilution of chromic chloride (0.033%) is added dropwise to a mixture of 25 µl of

ML34 at 400 µg/ml and 25 µl of packed SRBC. The mixture is then rotated for 1 h at room temperature, followed by three washes with PBS. The pellet is resuspended to 1% in PBS. The cells can be kept at 4 °C for up to 1 week.

Assay procedure: doubling dilutions of CSF are made on 96 well plates (flexible, U-shaped wells) in 25 µl volumes. MTSE and purified LAM-B dilutions are made as standards. ML34-coated red cells (25 µl) are added and haemagglutination reactions read after incubation for 1 h at 20 °C and overnight at 4 °C. Negative controls can include CSF with uncoated SRBC, PBS with coated SRBC and CSF with SRBC coated with an antibody of unrelated specificity. Haemagglutination can be observed with MTSE at 1 µg/ml.

Comments

Readers of this chapter, familiar with the routine diagnosis of tuberculosis, will recognise that as yet there is no accepted, fully evaluated serodiagnostic test for the disease. The methods described here must therefore be judged on their merits as potential assay systems. The results obtained thus far from the SACT-RIA assay suggest it has potential but requires further evaluation, particularly on smear-negative patients. The direct binding assay using purified antigens and the antigen trapping assays are all in their infancy and merit further investigations.

References

CHANDRAMUKI, A., ALLEN, P. R. J., KEEN, M. & IVANYI, J. 1985 Detection of mycobacterial antigen and antibodies in the cerebrospinal fluid of patients with tuberculous meningitis. *Journal of Medical Microbiology* **20**, 239–247.
COATES, A. R. M., ALLEN, B. W., HEWITT, J., IVANYI, J. & MITCHISON, D. A. 1981 Antigenic diversity of *M. tuberculosis* and *M. bovis* detected by means of monoclonal antibodies. *Lancet* ii, 167–169.
FRAKER, P. J. & SPECK, J. C. 1978 Protein and cell membrane iodinations with a sparingly soluble chloramide (Iodogen). *Biochemical and Biophysical Research Communications* **80**, 849–857.
GRANGE, J. M. 1984 The humoral immune response in tuberculosis: its nature, biological role and diagnostic usefulness. In *Advances in Tuberculosis Research, the Serology of Tuberculosis and BCG vaccination,* 21 ed. Fox, W., Grosset, J. & Styblo, K. pp. 1–78. Basel: S. Karger.
HEWITT, J., COATES, A. R. M., MITCHISON, D. A. & IVANYI, J. 1982 The use of murine monoclonal antibodies without purification of antigen in the serodiagnosis of tuberculosis. *Journal of Immunological Methods* **55**, 205–211.
HOEPPNER, V. H., JACKETT, P. S., BECK, J. S., KARDJITO, T., GRANGE, J. M. & IVANYI, J. 1978 Appraisal of the monoclonal antibody-based competition test for the serology of tuberculosis in Indonesia. *Serodiagnosis and Immunotherapy* **1**, 69–77.
HUNTER, S. W., GAYLORD, H. & BRENNAN, P. J. 1986 Structure and antigenicity of the phosphorylated lipopolysaccharide antigens from the leprosy and tubercle baccilli. *Biological Chemistry* **261**, 12345–12351.

IVANYI, J., KRAMBOVITIS, E. & KEEN, M. 1983 Evaluation of a monoclonal antibody (TB72) based serological test for tuberculosis. *Clinical and Experimental Immunology* **54**, 337–345.

IVANYI, J., MORRIS, J. A. & KEEN, M. 1985 Studies with monoclonal antibodies to mycobacteria. In *Monoclonal Antibodies Against Bacteria* ed. Macario, A. J. L. & Macario, E. C. pp. 59–90. London: Academic Press.

PRAPUTPITTAYA, K. & IVANYI, J. 1985 Detection of an antigen (MY4) common to *M. tuberculosis* and *M. leprae* by 'tandem' immunoassay. *Journal of Immunological Methods* **79**, 149–157.

RIDLEY, D. S. & JOPLING, W. H. 1966 Classification of leprosy according to immunity. A five-group system. *International Journal of Leprosy* **34**, 255–273.

SCOTT, M. L., THORNLEY, M. J., COOMBS, R. R. A. & BRADWELL, A. R. 1981 Measurement of human serum IgE and IgA by reverse passive antiglobulin haemagglutination. *International Archives of Allergy and Applied Immunology* **64**, 222–229.

SEVIER, E. D., DAVID, G. S., MARDNIS, J., DESMOND, W. J., BARTHOLOMEW, R. M. & WANG, R. 1981 Monoclonal antibodies in clinical immunology. *Clinical Chemistry* **27**, 1797–1806.

SINHA, S., SENGUPTA, U., RAMU, G. & IVANYI, J. 1983 A serological test for leprosy based on competitive inhibition of monoclonal antibody binding to the MY2a determinant of *Mycobacterium leprae*. *Transactions of the Royal Society of Tropical Medicine and Hygiene* **77**, 869–871.

SINHA, S., SENGUPTA, U., RAMU, G. & IVANYI, J. 1985 Serological survey of leprosy and control subjects by a monoclonal antibody-based immunoassay. *International Journal of Leprosy* **53**, 33–38.

SOOS, M. & SIDDLE, K. 1982 Characterization of monoclonal antibodies directed against human thyroid stimulating hormone. *Journal of Immunological Methods* **51**, 57–68.

UOTILA, M., RUOSLAHTI, E. & ENGVALL, E. 1981 Two-site sandwich enzyme immunoassay with monoclonal antibodies to human alpha-fetoprotein. *Journal of Immunological Methods* **42**, 11–15.

YOUNG, D., KENT, L., REES, A., LAMB, J. & IVANYI, J. 1986 Immunological activity of a 38 kilodalton protein purified from *Mycobacterium tuberculosis*. *Infection and Immunity* **54**, 177–183.

The Avidin–Biotin Technique in Immunocytochemical Staining

G. Coghill, J. Swanson Beck, J. H. Gibbs and R. S. Fawkes

Department of Pathology, Ninewells Hospital and Medical School, The University, Dundee DD1 9SY

Introduction

The invention of the fluorescent antibody technique (immunofluorescence) by Coons *et al.* (1941) was an important turning point in biological science, since for the first time it made possible the localization of antigens in tissues at a histological or cytological level. Subsequently, the range of macromolecules that can be identified has been limited only by the capacity of the immunologist to provide specific antisera: such polyclonal antibodies have limitations in specificity and the introduction of the monoclonal antibody technique (Kohler & Milstein, 1976) has made available a wide range of reagents specific for individual epitopes on many antigens.

This original immunofluorescence method suffered from the disadvantage of requiring a fluorescent microscope and darkened room for examination of the specimens. Moreover, the specimens were not permanent due to fading of the fluorescent ligand during microscopical examination and storage: such specimen fading can be minimized by using specialized mounting media (Johnson & Araujo, 1981), but the major problem of visualization of other tissue components during fluorescence microscopy has not been satisfactorily overcome.

Tinctorial dyes can be conjugated to antibodies but these are very insensitive reagents and the only practicable alternative for localization in tissues has been histochemical methods for detection of enzymes conjugated to antisera or purified immunoglobulins (Nakane & Pierce, 1966): the most successful enzymes for antibody labelling have been horseradish peroxidase (EC no 1.11.1.7), alkaline phosphatase derived from the small intestine (EC no 3.1.3.1), glucose oxidase (EC no 1.1.3.4) and β galactosidase derived from bacteria (EC no 3.2.1.23). The main criteria for the selection of an enzyme are high stability at room temperature, high specific activity and maintenance of its activity after coupling.

Immunological Techniques
in Microbiology

The original technique developed by Coons consisted of treating the tissue with the labelled immunoglobulin fraction from the specific antiserum (direct technique), but this was relatively insensitive and had the great disadvantage that each antiserum had to be conjugated to fluorescein before use. These difficulties were largely overcome by first treating the tissue with antiserum raised in one species to allow attachment of the antibody and, after washing away the excess serum, by staining the attached antibody with a fluorescein-conjugated antiserum to immunoglobulin raised in another species (indirect technique): the double layer results in considerable amplification and stronger staining intensity. Moreover, a single labelled second antibody can be used with a battery of first layer antisera.

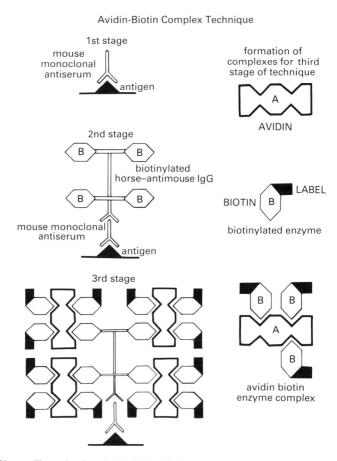

FIG. 1. Diagram illustrating the principle behind the biotin–avidin technique for molecular bridging in immunocytochemistry.

In subsequent development, emphasis was placed on improving sensitivity by increasing the number of layers in the staining procedure (but each additional layer made it more time-consuming and increased the extent of non-specific staining). The most efficient method so far devised involves conjugation of biotin to the immunoglobulin and attachment of the labelling molecule to avidin.

Avidin (molecular weight 67 000) is a glycoprotein constituent of egg white with histone-like characteristics: biotin is a small water-soluble vitamin. Each molecule of avidin can bind four molecules of biotin with very high affinity ($K_A 10^{-15} M^{-1}$) and the complex is stable even to high pH and to exposure to protein denaturing agents, proteolytic enzymes and organic solvents. Biotin can be readily conjugated to many proteins and a range of marker substances, such as enzymes and fluorescent dyes, can be combined with avidin without diminishing its capacity to bind biotin: these properties make the avidin–biotin technique a near ideal method for molecular bridging in immunocytochemistry (Fig. 1) (Warnke & Levy, 1980; Hsu *et al.*, 1981). The avidin–biotin system has also been used in the ELISA assay, nucleic acid hybridization (southern blots), protein detection (western blots) and in immunoaffinity techniques.

Streptavidin (molecular weight 60 000) is a protein component of *Streptomyces avidinii* with generally similar properties to avidin. Since it lacks the oligosaccharide residues (present on the avidin), it is less prone to give 'non-specific' attachment to tissue lectins (p. 101). In practice, Streptavidin can be used in exactly the same manner as avidin (Coggi *et al.*, 1986). The practical methods described in detail below have been selected because we have found these methods to be reliable in our laboratory.

Methods

Specimen preparation

While the techniques described here are applicable to material prepared in various ways, such as smears from centrifuged deposits, cytocentrifuge smears and touch or imprint preparations, the greater part of our work has been carried out on sections from frozen tissue samples which have been cut on a cryostat.

The cryostat consists of a refrigerated cabinet maintained at -20 °C, containing a microtome for sectioning tissues. To maintain the low temperatures the microtome controls (specimen advance and section thickness) are placed outside the cabinet. Most of the machines on the market (e.g. Reichert Jung, Bright Instruments Co. Ltd, and Slee Medical Equipment Ltd) perform satisfactorily: we have found the Slee models hard wearing, economical and reliable. The sections are cut with a disposable blade (Miles Scientific) and their natural tendency to curl is prevented by the use of an antiroll plate (Fig. 2). This is a glass plate coated with PTFE to prevent the sections sticking to it. A strip of Sellotape is folded over each side of the

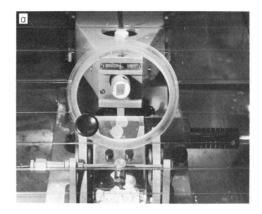

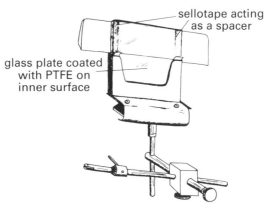

sellotape acting
as a spacer

glass plate coated
with PTFE on
inner surface

FIG. 2(a). Photograph of (Slee Medical Equipment, Ltd) cryostat showing section cutting of fresh frozen tissue. (b) Diagram illustrating the construction of an anti-roll plate; this is provided on most commercial instruments.

plate so that a gap is created between the plate and the knife. This gap, if correctly aligned against the knife, allows the section to slide through and prevents it curling.

To achieve good quality sections free from artefact certain conditions must be met. The tissue must be as fresh as possible and the freezing must be done quickly (less than 30 s), since the tissue will be distorted by ice crystal formation if the freezing process is prolonged. There are several alternative methods for snap-freezing tissue (Fig. 3) each with some advantages.

1 Solid carbon dioxide ('Dry-ice') and acetone. The tissue is attached to a metal cryostat chuck (Slee Medical Equipment Ltd) using 'OCT' gum (Raymond Lamb) ensuring correct orientation. The chuck is gently immersed, avoiding splashing, in a slurry of acetone with fragmented solid carbon dioxide. Care must be taken to

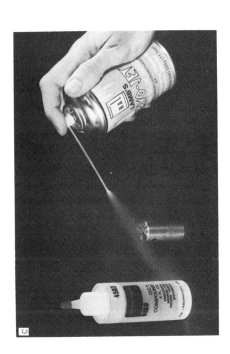

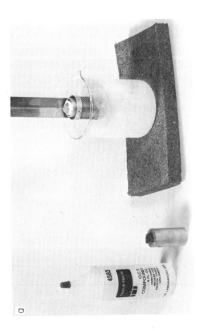

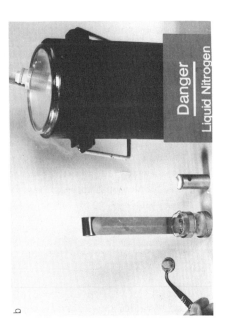

Fig. 3. Photographs illustrating the three most commonly used methods for snap-freezing tissue: (a) acetone/dry-ice slurry; (b) liquid nitrogen; and (c) freezing spray 'Cryo-Jet'.

avoid contamination of the tissue with acetone, since this solvent can dissolve in tissue fluids and interfere with solid freezing; tissue so affected can be difficult to cut in the cryostat. This is the most commonly used technique in the laboratory and, with care, gives the rapid freezing essential to avoid ice crystal damage to the tissues.

2 Liquid nitrogen and isopentane. For this technique a small beaker of isopentane is cooled by immersion in a Dewar flask of liquid nitrogen. The temperature of the isopentane is gauged to be low enough for freezing when it acquires the viscosity of glycerol. The tissue is attached by 'OCT' gum to a cork disc, presoaked in water to ensure attachment, and then plunged into the cooled isopentane where instant freezing occurs. The cork disc with frozen tissue can be attached to a metal chuck with gum and then frozen by immersion in the liquid nitrogen. This technique gives extremely fast freezing and has the additional advantage that it allows removal of the tissue block on the cork disc for storage. Contact of tissue with isopentane does not modify its cutting properties. In many ways this is the most desirable method, but liquid nitrogen is not freely available in all laboratories.

3 Cryogenic spray (Dichlorodifluoromethane). For this technique 'OCT' gum is placed on a firmly held cryostat chuck which is then cooled by spraying with 'Cryo-Jet' (Raymond Lamb). The tissue is placed in the gum and freezing is completed with further bursts of spray. This is a very convenient technique giving rapid freezing which can be carried out quite easily within the laboratory or 'on site'.

Once the tissues have been frozen by one of the above methods the blocks must be stored in a deep-freeze at a temperature of at least $-20\,°C$. To avoid dessication of the tissues, they are sealed by stretching 'Parafilm' (Gallenkamp) over the top of the chuck and round the sides: alternatively, the surface can be covered with 'OCT' gum and refrozen. If desired, the tissues may be stored in liquid nitrogen.

Frozen sections of tissue are usually the method of choice, since chemical fixation and histological processing to paraffin wax or resins can destroy many of the antigens. For those antigens which survive these procedures, however, the avidin-biotin techniques provide an excellent method for their demonstration, particularly when the antigen content is reduced by processing so that a high degree of sensitivity is required to demonstrate its presence.

Section preparation

Sections are usually cut at 6 μm (but thicker or thinner sections may be required for special processes) on a cryostat and placed on slides coated with adhesive to ensure attachment. Several forms of adhesives can be used.

1 Gelatine. Slides are cleaned by soaking in 95% alcohol, then wiped dry, placed in slide carrying racks, dipped in a jar of 0.5% aqueous solution of warmed gelatin, drained on tissue paper and allowed to dry in a dust free cupboard.

2 Poly-L-lysine (Huang *et al.*, 1983). Slides are prepared as above but are coated by spreading a small amount of 0.01% poly-L-lysine (Sigma Chemical Co. Ltd) over the slide surface: this is best done by using a slide as a spreader.

3 Aminoalkylsilane (Rentrop *et al.*, 1986). Slides are prepared as for gelatin coating, placed in racks and dipped in a 2% solution of aminoalkylsilane in anhydrous acetone for 5 s. They are then rinsed in fresh anhydrous acetone and allowed to dry. The latter two adhesives are more troublesome to prepare but give better adhesion for sections and smears that are prone to detachment during staining.

It is often desirable to stain a number of related sections on the same slide with different antisera for convenience in reading and to reduce subsequent problems of storage. It is possible to do this using multispot slides (Fig. 4) by the following method. The slides are pre-coated with Teflon leaving round clear 'windows' for section attachment: when applied carefully, the serological reagents will not spread from one test area to another during staining. Such slides can be purchased (Henley) or can be prepared in-house simply by placing drops of glycerol at the chosen 'window' areas and then spraying the slides with an aerosol of Teflon (McKay & Lynn). After drying, the glycerol is washed off leaving an area free of the water-repellent coating.

If difficulties are encountered in cutting the tissues on the cryostat, then sectioning may be improved by spraying the surface of the tissue with 'Cryo-Jet' (Raymond Lamb). This lowers the temperature, hardens the tissue and can allow better quality sections to be cut. If, however, the block is still too soft to cut properly, it can be thawed in 5% glycerol, cooled at 0 °C and left to soak for 15 min, before

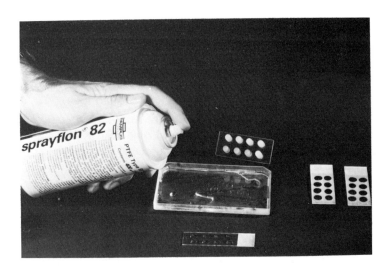

FIG. 4. Illustration of simple apparatus for preparation of multispot slides in the laboratory.

refreezing by one of the recommended methods. This treatment improves the cutting of sections without damaging the antigens (Coghill *et al.*, 1985) and can be used on fresh tissues before the initial freezing to improve preservation.

Sections can be stored for limited periods in slide racks or trays in a deep-freeze at -20 °C, but they are better sealed in boxes with silica gel to absorb moisture. Frozen sections should be allowed to return to room temperature before opening the boxes to avoid condensation on the surface.

Section handling procedures

Identification of the slides can be done by several methods. If plain glass slides are used, then a diamond pen must be used to scribe the identification on the same side as the specimen. The use of end frosted glass slides allows identification by 'lead' pencil and is the method preferred. Felt marker pens are quite unsuitable because the writing usually becomes illegible during the staining procedure.

To ensure that antiserum is placed on the area of the slide where the tissue section is attached, the underside of the slide is scribed with a diamond pen to produce a small circle around the section. This makes for easier visualization since the section often becomes very translucent after treatment with serum or washing. In Multispot slides, the section area is clearly delineated, but a plan is usually required to show which antisera have been applied to the individual areas.

The immunological staining reactions are carried out by laying the slides, section uppermost, on glass rods in long plastic trays: suitable trays can be purchased from Slee Medical Equipment Ltd or made up in the laboratory (Fig. 5(a)) and are then covered with plastic lids. The humidity in the tray must be kept high to minimize evaporation from the small volume of reagent applied during incubation: this is achieved by either adding a small amount of water to the tray or by laying moist tissue paper in its base. Buffer washes are performed by placing the slides in racks and immersing them in jars or bowls of buffer (Fig. 5(b)).

It is essential that the slides are wiped free of excess washing buffer solution before applying the subsequent reagent. This is best done by using an absorbent rag or paper tissue to mop up all fluid surrounding the tissue section. If this procedure is neglected, then the reagents may be overdiluted, producing weak or false-negative reactions. Care, however, must be taken to avoid complete drying of the sections at any stage in the staining procedure, since this can denature antigen or damage the histological or cytological structure due to exposure to hypertonic conditions.

Methods for section staining

Sections must be dried for at least 2 h after cutting otherwise there is a real risk that they will lift off the slide during staining. Thereafter the sections should be fixed to preserve cell morphology and antigenicity: acetone is the most widely-used fixative

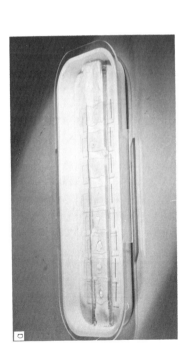

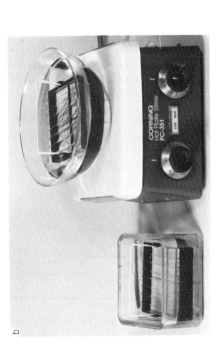

Fig. 5. Apparatus used in avidin–biotin immunocytochemical staining: (a) slide incubation moist chamber; (b) slide washing apparatus; and (c) commercial kit.

but for particular antigens acetone/methanol, acetone/chloroform or acetone/ methanol/formalin may prove superior. It is usual to allow the slides to dry so that the volatile protein-precipitating fixative is totally removed before the antiserum or monoclonal antibody is added. If, however, alkaline phosphatase is selected as the enzyme marker, drying of the tissue should be avoided and the slide rinsed in phosphate buffered saline (PBS) after fixation. Treatment for non-specific staining or removal of endogenous peroxidase (details of both are given later) can be applied at this stage. The duration of washing in buffer solution is not critical and these stages can be timed to suit the convenience of the working of the laboratory: in practice, we use brief immersions in two separate buffer baths, 3 min in each.

Optimal dilution of the first stage antiserum or monoclonal antibody must be determined empirically in preliminary experiments. With a new system we usually start from a dilution of 1/40, but the working dilution with various commercial reagents has varied within the range 1/5 to 1/2500. It is noteworthy that the greater sensitivity of the avidin–biotin system, compared with the indirect technique, often allows a first layer reagent to be used more economically at considerably greater dilution.

In most of our recent work we have used mouse monoclonal antibodies. Consequently, the second stage reagent is biotinylated polyclonal antimouse-Ig serum and we have found the Vectastain reagents (Seralab) very reliable and economical: the anti-IgG cross-reacts satisfactorily with IgM monoclonals in the first stage, but the anti-IgM is effectively monospecific. We have found that it is more economical to make up 1 ml of the diluted reagent by adding 5 µl biotinylated anti-IgG to 1000 µl PBS (rather than making up 10 ml as recommended) at each staining session, since this gives enough to treat 10–25 sections, depending on section size: if a section is very large, it is possible to apply a small drop of the expensive reagent and spread it out by carefully layering a clean coverslip on the surface to give a thin layer and to restrict evaporation.

The third stage reagent (avidin–biotin complex, ABC) comes in two solutions. It is essential that solution A (labelled 'avidin') and solution B (labelled 'biotinylated enzyme') are mixed and allowed to complex for at least 30 min at room temperature, following in detail the manufacturer's instructions. However, as with the second stage reagent, we prepare only enough for immediate use, usually 10 µl solution A is added to 1000 µl PBS and carefully mixed before addition of 10 µl solution B and remixing.

Details of a simple protocol for staining sections are given in Table 1.

Histochemical development of enzyme label

The horseradish peroxidase label is visualized with standard methods which give a choice of final colour complex (Van Noorden, 1986). Peroxidase catalyses the reduction of hydrogen peroxide to water by electron transfer from the substrate salt

TABLE 1. *Protocol for immunocytochemical staining*

1. Cut 6–8 μm frozen sections and attach to adhesive-coated slides
2. Allow to dry for at least 2 h: scribe identification and mark position of section
3. Fix in acetone at room temperature for 10–20 min
4. Allow section to dry
5. Apply monoclonal antibody to section and leave for 30 min
6. Wash briefly in PBS
7. Apply biotinylated second antibody for 30 min
8. Wash briefly in PBS
9. Apply ABC (avidin–biotin complex) for 45 min
10. Wash briefly in PBS
11. Develop enzyme; if peroxidase, follow with 1% copper sulphate
12. Wash in water
13. Counterstain nuclei with Mayer's haematoxylin 30 s
14. Wash in water
15. 'Blue' nuclei in Scott's Tap Water Substitute
16. Wash in water
17. Mount in suitable medium (dehydrate and clear if BPS used)

to give a coloured end-product, which is usually insoluble or at worst partially insoluble, at the site of the enzyme marker.

The commonest method uses diaminobenzidine (DAB) (Graham & Karnovsky, 1966): we prefer this method because it gives a dark brown end-product to contrast with counter-stain and it is insoluble in alcohol so that the sections can be mounted in BPS plastic mountant: this mounting media has a refractive index of 1.52, closely similar to that for glass, so the microscopic image is very bright and has good definition of the specimen. BPS (Raymond Lamb) is easily dispensed from metal ('toothpaste') tubes (Adelphi Tubes) and sets within a few hours.

The colour of the DAB reaction product in peroxidase staining can be improved by adding 0.01 M imidazole to the buffer used to dissolve the DAB (Straus, 1982). Treatment of the sections with 1% copper sulphate in isotonic saline after completion of the DAB reaction makes the histochemical staining more intense (Becton Dickinson Source Book, 1985).

Many other chemicals can be used as alternatives (Table 2), if other colours are desired e.g., aminoethylcarbazole (AEC) (Graham *et al.*, 1965) and chloronaphthol (CN) (Nakane, 1968), which give a red (AEC) or blue (CN) final end-product respectively, but these substrates have the serious disadvantage that, being alcohol soluble, they can be mounted only in water-based mounting media. We use Highman's modification (Raymond Lamb) of Apathys medium, which has a refractive index of 1.52, which is higher than most aqueous mounting media but it nevertheless suffers from the disadvantage of being impermanent, sticky and slow setting.

TABLE 2. *Histochemical methods for development of immunocytochemical staining*

Substrate	Colour	Mounting media	Counterstain	Advantages/disadvantages
Label—horseradish peroxidase				
Diaminobenzidine (DAB)	Brown	DPX (resinous)	Mayers haematoxylin (colour blue)	Permanent—strong colour—suitable for double staining
Aminoethylcarbazole (AEC)	Red	Highmans (aqueous)	Mayers haematoxylin (colour blue)	Impermanent—gives good cytoplasmic staining
Chloronaphthol (CN)	Blue	Highmans (aqueous)	Kernechtrot (colour red)	Impermanent—suitable for double staining with DAB or AEC
Label—alkaline phosphatase				
Fast Red TR + naphthol AS MX phosphate	Red	Highmans (aqueous)	Mayers haematoxylin (colour blue)	Impermanent—good strong colour—suitable for surface markers on smears and imprints
Fast Blue BB + naphthol AS MX phosphate	Blue	Highmans (aqueous)	Kernechtrot (colour red)	Impermanent—good contrast with red end product in double staining
Hexazotised dyes (HPR/HNF + naphthol AS MX phosphate)	Red	DPX (resinous)	Mayers haematoxylin (colour blue)	Better than Fast Red TR for surface markers in tissue sections—excellent contrast with DAB in permanent preparations
Fast Red TR + sodium α-naphthyl phosphate	Brown	Highmans (aqueous)	Mayers haematoxylin (colour blue)	Impermanent brown colour particulate

Other less suitable aqueous media that can be used include the original Apathys Mountant or Kaisers Glycerin Jelly (both available from Raymond Lamb).

Alkaline phosphatase catalyses the hydrolysis of phosphate esters and in histochemical staining substituted naphthol compounds such as naphthol AS-BI or MX phosphate are degraded to release the 'primary reaction product' (PRP) which immediately combines with a diazonium or hexazonium salt to form a 'final reaction product' (FRP) containing the appropriate diazo or hexazo dye (Mason & Sammons, 1978; Mason, 1985). The FRP from hexazotised new fuchsin and naphthol AS-BI phosphate is extremely insoluble in water. Various diazonium salts, such as Fast Red TR or Fast Blue BB, can be substituted to give an appropriate final colour (Table 2). The end-product of all these methods is insoluble in water, but fairly soluble in alcohol or other histological solvents, consequently the preparations must be mounted in a water-based mounting medium. If a permanent preparation in non-aqueous BPS mountant is required, then naphthol AS-BI or MX phosphate with hexazotised pararosaniline or new fuchsin must be used to produce a strong red colour. All chemicals for these histochemical methods are available from Sigma Chemical Co Ltd.

Laboratory hazards in histochemical staining

All the special chemicals used for histochemical staining are considered hazardous (Griswold et al., 1968): DAB and AEC are potential carcinogens so should be handled with due safety precautions, but recent reviews (Tubbs & Sheibani, 1982) have suggested that DAB is less dangerous than was previously thought (Weisberger et al., 1978).

The trays used for histochemical staining can be decontaminated by treating them with 0.1% sodium hypochlorite for at least 15 min. Disposable gloves must be worn during section handling which should properly take place in a fume cupboard with effective extraction and this should be lined with absorbent paper ('Benchkote', Gallenkamp). Waste, including gloves, plastic pipettes and universal bottles should be placed in a polythene bag, tied at the neck and incinerated.

To reduce the handling required for DAB, we routinely make up large amounts (500 ml), aliquot the solution into 10 ml volumes and store these in plastic universal bottles in the deep-freeze at -20 °C. Running hot water is used to thaw the DAB solution before the addition of the hydrogen peroxide (10 μl to each tube of DAB).

Non-specific staining

In concept, the immunocytochemical techniques consist of the application of a series of serological reactions to localize an enzyme marker at the site of the target antigen with subsequent localization by an enzyme histochemical reaction. In practice non-specific staining can arise in various ways from effects at different stages of the staining procedure (Table 3).

Tissue: all tissues contain enzymes and it is generally inadvisable to choose an enzyme marker with an activity similar to that of an enzyme known to be abundant in the tissue. Endogenous peroxidase is found in macrophages and polymorphs, and certain iron-containing pigments (such as haemoglobin and myoglobin) can catalyse an analogous reaction: the advantages of peroxidase as a marker are great and it is often worth the trouble of eliminating the artefact of endogenous staining by one of the three available methods.

1 Sections are treated for 30 min with absolute ethanol containing 0.5% hydrogen peroxide and 0.074% hydrochloric acid (Straus, 1971).

TABLE 3. *Types, causes and remedies of non-specific staining*

Type of staining	Cause	Remedy
Intensely dark staining cells when using peroxidase as a label	Cells containing endogenous peroxidase e.g. macrophages	Block endogenous enzyme: use alternative label
Positive cells and tissue components when using alkaline phosphatase as a label	Cells containing endogenous alkaline phosphatase e.g. polymorph neutrophils	Block endogenous enzyme: use alternative label
Positive staining in muco-substances and mast cells	Avidin reacting non-specifically with oligosaccharides and mucosubstances	Raise pH of buffer for ABC reaction: use streptavidin
Generalized or focal background	Non specific non-immunological reaction with either primary or secondary antisera	Dilute antisera by titration for optimal staining contrast: absorb with tissue powder or homogenate or with activated charcoal: use fetal calf serum: use washing buffer with different pH
Unexpected reaction with other tissue components	Epitope of immunizing antigen located in unrelated antigens	Check antisera on a wide range of tissues

2 Heyderman & Neville (1977) have recommended that sections be treated with:

7.5% aqueous hydrogen peroxide	—5 min
washed in running water	—5 min
2.4% aqueous periodic acid	—5 min
washed in running water	—5 min
freshly prepared 0.03% aqueous sodium borohydride	—3 min
washed in running water	—5 min

3 1 mM phenylhydrazine in phosphate buffered saline at 37 °C for 60 min (Jasani *et al.*, 1983).

Some antigens do not survive the first two methods and for these, the third method may prove satisfactory. With a very labile antigen, another approach is to apply the first antibody layer and then to block endogenous peroxidase before completion of the immunocytochemical staining. It is even possible to use the peroxidase techniques without any attempt at blocking of endogenous peroxidase: careful comparison between sections receiving the whole staining procedure and controls (lacking the final avidin–peroxidase layer) may permit the discrimination between endogenous and applied peroxidase activity.

Alkaline phosphatase does not usually present such great problems, but when the endogenous enzyme is abundant (as in macrophages and endothelium) it can be blocked by levamisole (Ponder & Wilkinson, 1981). Small intestinal alkaline phosphatase cannot be blocked in this way but the oxidative procedure for peroxidase (2 above) can block artefactual staining in this site (Bulman & Heyderman, 1982).

In other circumstances glucose oxidase or β galactosidase can produce less confusion, but these labelled enzymes are more expensive and the histochemical reaction product is less stable. To-date, we have always been able to localize antigens with either the peroxidase or alkaline phosphatase methods and we have not yet been forced to use the expensive glucose oxidase or β galactosidase reagents.

Serological reagents: monoclonal antibodies are monospecific for the appropriate epitopes, consequently these should rarely give rise to true non-specific staining (but other problems may arise, see below). By contrast, polyclonal antisera are never monospecific since these will contain antibodies reflecting the previous immunological experience of the donor animal: affinity purification can reduce this cause of unwanted staining, but not all commercial products are marketed in this form. Moreover, animal sera may contain various macromolecules that combine non-immunologically, but with high avidity, to tissue components (Mayersbach & Schubert, 1960). Such causes of non-specific staining should be recognized by proper selection of controls. When encountered, these imperfections can usually be overcome by classical serological absorption methods using tissue homogenates, acetone-dried tissue powders or activated charcoal in an empirical manner (Beck & Currie, 1967).

An alternative method for elimination of troublesome non-specific staining of the tissue background involves pre-treatment of the sections for 30 min prior to immunological staining with a solution of either (1) 1% bovine serum albumin with 1% fetal calf serum (or unconjugated serum) and 0.1% sodium azide in phosphate buffered saline; or (2) unconjugated serum. In practice using the ABC kits, we have had no major problems related to these forms of non-specific reaction.

Avidin: this protein is highly specific for biotin, but it can under certain circumstances show a lesser affinity for tissue muco-substances, mast cells (Bussolati & Gugliotti, 1983; Tharp *et al.*, 1985) and certain lectins, due to its oligosaccharide content. This type of non-specific staining can usually be minimized by pretreatment of the section with high pH (usually 9.4) buffer. Streptavidin (Amersham International) does not contain these oligosaccharides (Bonnard *et al.*, 1984) and is effective as a biotin-binding enzyme carrier molecule.

Tissue biotin: some tissues such as liver, breast and kidney may bind enzyme-labelled avidin through their endogenous biotin content. Such non-specific staining can be minimized by treatment of the tissue with unlabelled avidin followed by free biotin (Wood & Warnke, 1981) to block the tissue before the immunocytochemical staining is started: there are thus no free tissue binding groups available when the avidin–biotin technique is carried out.

Specificity of monoclonal antibodies

When available, monoclonal antibodies should be used as the primary reagent in immunological staining because each is monospecific for a unique epitope on the antigen under consideration. It must, however, be remembered that similar epitopes may occasionally be found on other macromolecules. Not surprisingly, some epitopes are shared between closely related sources, e.g., some monoclonal antibodies to *M. leprae* react equally well with similar affinity to the corresponding molecules in *M. tuberculosis*. However, epitope sharing of a type that could not reasonably be predicted is occasionally encountered, e.g., the MC2 monoclonal antibody to human granulocyte cell surface (McCarthy *et al.*, 1985) cross reacts strongly with human astrocytic glial fibres, and the commercially available 'LEU4' and 'LEU7' prepared against human lymphoid cells (Becton Dickinson) cross-react with Purkinje cells (Garson *et al.*, 1982) in the cerebellum and neuro–endocrine granules (Shioda *et al.*, 1984) respectively. It must be remembered that such reactions are not artefacts and they are not nonspecific in immunological terms since they arise from the chance appearance of similar regions of molecular structure in otherwise unrelated macromolecules. Because of these difficulties, individual macromolecules must be conclusively identified by the presence of clusters of differentiation antigens (Bernard *et al.*, 1984): this approach has been most widely applied to the definition of lymphoid cells but will soon be applied to other fields of research to give unique identification.

Selection of controls (Summarized in Table 4)

It is our usual practice to substitute buffered saline for the monoclonal antibody in the first stage of the immunocytochemical staining. This allows us to check whether the detection system or the tissue section can be the cause of non-specific staining. The second essential control is to replace the specific monoclonal antibody with an irrelevant or 'nonsense' mouse monoclonal antibody, prepared under similar conditions to the specific reagent (i.e., culture supernatant or ascitic fluid) and diluted to comparable immunoglobulin concentration: this control should not give

TABLE 4.   *Control procedures*

1. Tissue containing and lacking specific antigen
2. Omission of first layer antiserum and substitution of buffer solution, nonimmune or preimmune sera, or unrelated antisera
3. Absorption of antisera with specific and unrelated antigens
4. Omission of biotinylated peroxidase

any staining if the detection system is clear. If this control fails, a logical approach to elimination of the cause of non-specific staining should allow the investigator to achieve specific results. It is of course essential to have a tissue substrate that naturally contains (or has had artificially added) specific antigen and it is desirable to have tissue lacking the antigen as a negative control.

The same principles apply with polyclonal antisera, but these require greater care because they frequently contain unexpected antibodies (e.g., any animal which has been immunized with Freund's Complete Adjuvant will incidentally have antibodies to mycobacteria in addition to those towards the immunizing antigen). Such sera will usually require control non-immune (or, even better, pre-immune) serum and the antisera should become negative after specific absorption but remain positive when absorbed by an unrelated antigen.

Counterstaining of sections

It is desirable, although not essential, to stain the cell nuclei a different colour from that of the antigen localization. This allows the sites of the positive reaction to be related to the tissue structure (Fig. 6).

Our normal practice is to treat the section after immunocytochemical staining with Mayer's Haematoxylin for 30 s and then with an alkaline solution, Scotts Tap Water Substitute, for 2 min. This results in the nuclei of the cells being blue and

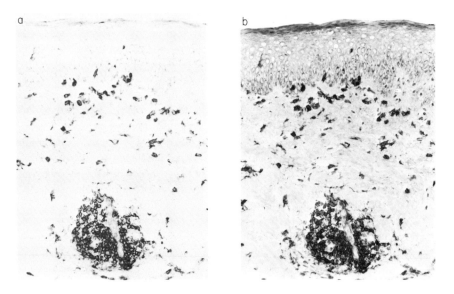

FIG. 6. Illustration of the value of a nuclear counterstain for localization of the microanatomical site of immunocytochemical staining: (a) no counterstain; and (b) Mayer's haematoxylin counterstain.

this colour contrasts well with specific red or brown staining of antigen by DAB, AEC, Fast Red TR or HNF/HPR. When the antigen sites are shown as a final blue colour with CN or Fast Blue B, counterstaining with the red dye Kernechtrot for 2 min will provide a contrasting colour in the cell nuclei. For specialized purposes, a wide range of histological stains are available so that immunocytochemical localization can be attributed to many selected histological features.

Sections for aqueous mounting are washed and then mounted in Highman's Media. Sections for mounting in BPS are dehydrated in two changes of 95% ethanol, two changes of absolute ethanol, a mixture of absolute alcohol and xylene and three changes of xylene.

Photography

The modern photomicroscope with its corrected matching optics and sophisticated metering systems is potentially a very efficient instrument, but high quality photomicrographs can only be produced with a proper understanding of the principles of operation. The manufacturers' manuals are generally well written and the instructions should be followed carefully: the condenser must be centred and Köhler illumination set up for each chosen objective.

Colour transparencies are relatively easy to prepare. There is a wide choice of 35 mm colour reversal films suitable for photomicrography. Kodak Ektachrome EPN 100, balanced for daylight, has consistently given good results in our hands, provided that the colour temperature of the microscope lamp is balanced to that of the film with appropriate blue filters.

It is more difficult to prepare good quality black and white prints for illustration of manuscripts. Most photomicroscopes use a 35 mm camera format, consequently the negative must be enlarged at least four-fold for printing. It is therefore essential to use a fine grain film with high resolving power and inherent high contrast to reproduce the very poorly stained background. We have found that Kodak Technical Pan Film 2415 gives good records of immunoperoxidase stained preparations: the contrast can be adjusted by altering the developer solution and the film speed rating. A useful trial may be made with a film speed set at 50 ASA, developing for 8 min at 20 °C in Kodak HC110 developer diluted 1:19 (Kodak HC110 comes as a highly concentrated solution which is initially diluted 1:3 to give a stock solution for further dilution as required). This 'one shot' development technique gives very consistent results, and should produce clear negatives with a contrast index of approximately 1.0, printing on normal or soft bromide papers.

The gold brown reaction product with DAB can be enhanced by using a blue filter, such as the Kodak Wratten 38A filter, available in gelatine squares which can be mounted between two $2 \times 2''$ coverglasses. Since this type of filter is placed in the light path below the section, expensive optical filters are unnecessary and the metering system will automatically compensate for their use. If the nuclei are

TABLE 5. *Use of colour filters in photomicrography*

Peroxidase developer reagents	Reaction product colour	Filter colour
Diaminobenzidine	Golden brown	Blue
3-Amino-9-ethylcarbazole	Red-brown	Green
4-Chloro-1-naphthol	Blue	Yellow or orange

stained blue with haemalum the 38A filter will help to render them as a light grey on the final print, avoiding any confusion with the black positive DAB staining (Fig. 6). The contrast of other coloured reaction products can be increased by using complementary colour filters (Table 5).

Quantitation of immunocytochemical staining

There can be considerable variations in intensity of immunocytochemical staining at different points within a section or between samples. Nevertheless it is not practicable to quantitate with any degree of precision the amount of the corresponding antigen at a locus because of the kinetic variations in the reactions at the various stages of immunological and enzyme histochemical staining.

It is, however, reasonable to attempt to measure the numbers of cells bearing particular antigens: there are a variety of relatively simple histometric techniques available that involve 'point-counting' or related observations and do not require specialized apparatus (Beck & Anderson, 1987). More simple semiquantitative morphological assessments can be used to determine cell density and distribution from monochrome photomicrographs (Gibbs *et al.*, 1984). Such methods are applicable to many biological problems.

Appendix I

Formulae for preparation of reagents

Buffers

PHOSPHATE BUFFERED SALINE (PBS)

This is the commonest buffer used for rinsing sections and preparing dilutions of the immunological reagents.

Dipotassium hydrogen phosphate (K_2HPO_4)   —75.2 g
Sodium dihydrogen phosphate (NaH_2PO_4)   —14.8 g
Sodium chloride   —72 g
Distilled water   —10 litre

Tris buffered saline (TBS)

This is an alternative buffer to PBS which can sometimes help reduce non-specific background.

Tris   —12.1 g
Sodium chloride   —160 g
Distilled water   —20 litre
1 M HCl   —70 ml
Adjust pH to 7.6 with the addition of 1 M HCl

Peroxidase substrates

3,3–diaminobenzidine (dab)

This is the normal substrate salt used for peroxidase detection giving dark brown positivity.

3,3–Diaminobenzidine (DAB)   —5 mg
Phosphate buffered saline (PBS)   —10 ml

Add 10 μl of hydrogen peroxide (100 vol/30%) immediately before use. Incubate for 10 min at room temperature.

3–amino-9-ethylcarbazole (aec)

This substrate is used if a red positive result is required. Stock Solution: 0.4% AEC in dimethylformamide.

Incubating solution: Stock AEC   —0.5 ml
                      0.05 M acetate buffer pH 5.0   —9.5 ml
                      Hydrogen peroxide (30%)   —10 μl

Filter solution on to slides—incubate for 20–30 min at room temperature (times can be reduced by half at 37 °C).

4–chloro-1-naphthol (cn)

This substrate is used if blue end-product is required. Dissolve 40 mg CN in 0.2 ml absolute ethanol. Add (stirring constantly) 100 ml 0.05 M Tris buffer (TBS) pH 7.6 along with 50 μl of hydrogen peroxide (30%).
Filter solution on to slides—incubate for 20 min at room temperature (shorter times at temperatures up to 50 °C).

Alkaline phosphatase substrates

HEXAZOTIZED NEW FUCHSIN

This substrate is used if a permanent red end-product is desired

Naphthol AS–BI phosphate (free acid)	—10 mg
Dimethylformamide	—0.1 ml
0.05 M Tris buffer pH 8.7	—20 ml
1 M levamisole	—20 µl
4% sodium nitrite	—0.1 ml
5% new fuchsin (or Pararosaniline)	—0.04 ml

Add the nitrite solution to the new fuchsin in a glass beaker: mix and leave for 1 min (this is best done in a fume cupboard). Add the Tris buffer. (The Tris buffer is most easily made by diluting 0.2 M Tris. If this is done there is usually no need to estimate the pH of the solution as the pararosaniline solution will lower the pH to 8.7.) Add the levamisole. In a separate beaker dissolve the naphthol AS–BI phosphate in dimethylformamide (if the sodium salt is used it can be dissolved directly in the buffer). Mix the two solutions: check pH if required and filter on to slides. Incubate for 15–20 min at room temperature.

DIAZONIUM SALT (1)

These substrates are used if a red or blue end-product is desired

Naphthol AS–MX phosphate	—2 mg
Dimethylformamide	—0.2 ml
0.1 M Tris pH 8.2	—9.8 ml
1 M levamisole	—10 µl
Fast Red TR or Fast Blue BB	—10 mg

Dissolve the Naphthol AS–MX phosphate in dimethylformamide in a glass beaker. Add the Tris buffer and the levamisole. (This stock can be deep frozen at −20 °C.) Dissolve the appropriate diazonium salt in the substrate solution—check pH and filter onto slides. Incubate for 15–20 min at room temperature.

DIAZONIUM SALT (2)

This substrate is used for a red brown end-product

Sodium α naphthyl phosphate	—10 mg
0.2 M Tris	—10 ml
1 M levamisole	—10 µl
Fast Red TR	—10 mg

Dissolve the sodium α naphthyl phosphate in the Tris. Add the levamisole and the Fast Red TR. (Do not check pH.) Filter onto slides and incubate at room temperature for 10–20 min.

Appendix II

List of suppliers

Immunological reagents	*Accessory supplies*
Ortho Pharmaceuticals	Slee Medical Equipment Ltd
Becton Dickinson	Miles Scientific
Coulter Electronics	Henley
Dako	Adelphi Tubes
Serotec	Gallenkamp
Seralab	Raymond Lamb
Amersham International	Sigma Chemical Co. Ltd
	Chroma
	McKay & Lynn
	Bright Instrument Co. Ltd
	Reichert Jung U.K.

Essential source book

Linscott's Directory of Immunological and Biological Reagents. 4th Edn 1986–87. Available from Linscott's Directories, P.O. Box 55, East Grinstead, Sussex RH19 3YL, England.

References

BECK, J. S. & ANDERSON, J. M. 1987 Quantitative methods as an aid to diagnosis in histopathology. In *Recent Advances in Histopathology* ed. Anthony, P. P. & MacSween, R. N. M. Vol. 13 pp. 255–269. Edinburgh: Churchill Livingstone.

BECK, J. S. & CURRIE, A. R. 1967 Immunofluorescence localisation of growth hormone in the human pituitary gland and of a related antigen in the syncytiotrophoblast. *Vitamins and Hormones* 25, 89–211.

BECTON DICKINSON SOURCE BOOK 1985. California: Becton Dickinson Monoclonal Center, Inc.

BERNARD, A., BOUMSELL, L., DAUSSET, J., MILSTEIN, C. & SCHLOSSMAN, S. F. 1984 *Leucocyte Typing.* Berlin: Springer Verlag.

BONNARD, C., PAPERMASTER, D. S. & KRAEHENBUHL, J. P. 1984 The streptavidin–biotin bridge technique: application in light and electron microscope immunocytochemistry. In *Immunolabelling for Electron Microscopy* ed. Polak, J. & Varndell, I. M. pp. 95–111. Amsterdam: Elsevier Scientific Publishers.

BULMAN, A. S. & HEYDERMAN, E. 1982 Alkaline phosphatase for immunocytochemical labelling. Problems with endogenous activity. *Journal of Clinical Pathology* 34, 1349–1351.

BUSSOLATI, G. & GUGLIOTTI, P. 1983 Non specific staining of mast cells by avidin–biotin–peroxidase complexes (ABC). *Journal of Histochemistry and Cytochemistry* **31**, 1419–1421.

COGGI, G., DELL'ORTO, P. & VIALE, G. 1986 Avidin Biotin Methods. In *Immunocytochemistry Modern Methods and Applications* 2nd Edn. eds. Polak, J. M. & Van Noorden, S. pp. 54–70. Bristol: Wright.

COGHILL, G., GIBBS, J. H., LOWE, J. G. & BECK, J. S. 1985 Cryopreservation with glycerol during cryostat sectioning for localisation of lymphocytes and accessory cell phenotypic subsets in tissue biopsies. *Journal of Clinical Pathology* **38**, 840–842.

COONS, A. H., CREECH, H. J. & JONES, R. N. 1941 Immunological properties of an antibody containing a fluorescent group. *Proceedings of the Society for Experimental Biology and Medicine* **47**, 200–202.

GARSON, J. A., BEVERLEY, P. C. L., COAKHAM, H. B. & HARPER, E. I. 1982 Monoclonal antibodies against human T lymphocytes label Purkinje neurones of many species. *Nature* **298**, 375–377.

GIBBS, J. H., FERGUSON, J., BROWN, R. A., KENICER, K. J. A., POTTS, R. C., COGHILL, G. & BECK, J. S. 1984 Histometric study of the localisation of lymphocyte subsets and accessory cells in human Mantoux reactions. *Journal of Clinical Pathology* **37**, 1227–1234.

GRAHAM, R. C. & KARNOVSKY, M. J. 1966 The early stages of absorption of injected horseradish peroxidase in the proximal tubules of mouse kidney ultrastructural cytochemistry by a new technique. *Journal of Histochemistry and Cytochemistry* **14**, 291–302.

GRAHAM, R. C. JR., LUDHOLM, U. & KARNOVSKY, M. J. 1965 Cytochemical demonstration of peroxidase activity with 3-amino-9-ethyl-carbazole. *Journal of Histochemistry and Cytochemistry* **13**, 150–152.

GRISWOLD, D. P. JR., CASEY, A. E., WEISBURGER, E. U. & WEISBURGER, J. H. 1968 The carcinogenicity of multiple intragastric doses of aromatic and heterocyclic nitro or amino derivatives in young female Sprague-Dawley rats. *Cancer Research* **28**, 924–933.

HEYDERMAN, E. & NEVILLE, A. M. 1977 A shorter immunoperoxidase technique for the demonstration of carcinoembryonic antigen and other cell products. *Journal of Clinical Pathology* **30**, 138–140.

HSU, S. M., RAINE, L. & FANGER, H. 1981 Use of avidin–biotin–peroxidase complex (ABC) in immunoperoxidase techniques: a comparison between ABC and unlabelled antibody (PAP) procedures. *Journal of Histochemistry and Cytochemistry* **29**, 577–580.

HUANG, W., GIBSON, S. J., FACER, P., GU, J. & POLAK, J. M. 1983 Improved section adhesion for immunocytochemistry using high molecular weight polymers of L-lysine as a slide coating. *Histochemistry* **77**, 175–279.

JASANI, B., HALLAM, L. A., NEWMAN, G. R. & WILLIAMS, E. D. 1983 Non-deleterious inhibition of endogenous peroxidase in immunolocalisation studies involving the use of monoclonal antibodies. *Histochemical Journal* **15**, 1257–1258.

JOHNSON, G. D. & ARAUJO, G. M. DE C. N. 1981 A simple method of reducing the fading of immunofluorescence during microscopy. *Journal of Immunological Methods* **43**, 349–350.

KOHLER G. & MILSTEIN, C. 1976 Derivation of specific antibody producing tissue culture and tumour lines by cell fusion. *European Journal of Immunology* **6**, 511–519.

McCARTHY, N. C., SIMPSON, J. R. M., COGHILL, G. & KERR, M. A. 1985 Expression in normal adult, fetal, and neoplastic tissues of a carbohydrate differentiation antigen recognised by antigranulocyte mouse monoclonal antibodies. *Journal of Clinical Pathology* **38**, 521–529.

MASON, D. Y. 1985 Immunocytochemical labelling of monoclonal antibodies by the APAAP immunoalkaline phosphatase technique. In *Techniques in Immunocytochemistry* ed. Bullock, G. R. & Petrusz, P. pp. 25–40. London: Academic Press.

MASON, D. Y. & SAMMONS, R. 1978 Alkaline phosphatase and peroxidase for double immunoenzymatic labelling of cellular constituents. *Journal of Clinical Pathology* **31**, 454–460.

MAYERSBACH, H. & SCHUBERT, G. 1960 Immunological Methods III. The unspecific reaction between labelled serum and tissues in the immunohistological technique. *Acta Histochemica* **10**, 44–82.

NAKANE, P. K. 1968 Simultaneous localisation of multiple tissue antigens using the peroxidase-labelled antibody method: a study in pituitary glands of the rat. *Journal of Histochemistry and Cytochemistry* **16**, 557–560.

NAKANE, P. K. & PIERCE, G. B. JR. 1966 Enzyme labelled antibodies: preparation and application for the localisation of an antigen. *Journal of Histochemistry and Cytochemistry* 14, 929–931.

PONDER, B. A. & WILKINSON, M. M. 1981 Inhibition of endogenous tissue alkaline phosphatase with the use of alkaline phosphatase conjugate in immunochemistry. *Journal of Histochemistry and Cytochemistry* 29, 981–984.

RENTROP, M., KNAPP, B., WINTER, H. & SCHWEIZER, J. 1986 Aminoalkylsilane-treated glass slides as support for *in situ* hybridisation of keratin cDNA to frozen tissue sections under varying fixation and pretreatment conditions. *Histochemical Journal* 18, 271–276.

SHIODA, Y., NAGURA, H., TSUTSUMI, Y., SHIMAMURA, K. & TAMAOKI, N. 1984 Distribution of Leu7 (HNK-1) antigen in human digestive organs: an immunohistochemical study with monoclonal antibody. *Histochemical Journal* 16, 843–854.

STRAUS, W. 1971 Inhibition of peroxidase by methanol and methanol nitroferricyanide for use in immunoperoxidase procedures. *Journal of Histochemistry and Cytochemistry* 19, 682–688.

STRAUS, W. 1982 Imidazole increases the sensitivity of the cytochemical reaction for peroxidase with Diaminobenzidine at a neutral pH. *Journal of Histochemistry and Cytochemistry* 50, 491–493.

THARP, M. D., SEELIG, L. L., TIGELAAR, R. E. & BERGSTRESSER, P. R. 1985 Conjugated avidin binds to mast cell granules. *Journal of Histochemistry and Cytochemistry* 33, 27–32.

TUBBS, R. R. & SHEIBANI, K. 1982 Chromogens for immunohistochemistry. *Archives of Pathology and Laboratory Medicine* 106, 205.

VAN NOORDEN, S. 1986 Tissue preparation and immunostaining techniques for light microscopy. In *Immunocytochemistry Modern Methods and Applications*, 2nd Edn. ed. Polak, J. M. & Van Noorden, S. pp. 26–53. Bristol: Wright.

WARNKE, R. & LEVY, R. 1980 Detection of T and B cell antigens with hybridoma monoclonal antibodies: a biotin–avidin–horseradish peroxidase method. *Journal of Histochemistry and Cytochemistry* 28, 771–776.

WEISBURGER, E. K., RUSSFIELD, A. B., HOMBURGER, F., WEISBURGER, J. H., BOGER, E., VAN DONGEN, C. G. & CHU, K. C. 1978 Testing of twenty one environmental aromatic amines or derivatives for long term toxicity of carcinogenicity. *Journal of Environmental Pathology and Toxicology* 2, 325–350.

WOOD, G. S. & WARNKE, R. 1981 Suppression of endogenous avidin-binding activity in tissues and its relevance to biotin–avidin detection systems. *Journal of Histochemistry and Cytochemistry* 29, 1196–1204.

Immunogold Labelling of Fungal Enzymes

P. T. ATKEY AND D. A. WOOD

*Glasshouse Crops Research Institute, Worthing Road, Littlehampton, West Sussex
BN17 6LP*

Introduction

The cultivated mushroom *Agaricus bisporus* utilizes composted wheat straw as its
commercial growth substrate. Studies on the nutritional physiology of the organism
in both liquid and solid substrate culture show that a variety of extracellular
enzymes are produced, including both oxidases and hydrolases (Wood, 1984). The
most abundant extracellular enzyme in all growth media is an extracellular phenol
oxidase—a laccase.

Developmental studies show that the extractable activity of this enzyme
increases in parallel with mycelial biomass up to the stage of fruit body enlargement
(Wood & Goodenough, 1977; Wood, 1979). Beyond this stage activity declines
rapidly to about 10% of peak activity.

The enzyme has been purified from cultures grown in liquid media, and from
solid substrate grown cultures at two stages of morphogenesis, before and after fruit
development. Antibodies have been raised to all three enzyme preparations (Wood,
1980a, b). The enzymes detected in the different media and at the various stages
show some cross-reactions (identity) and some non-identity. Analytical studies
show the enzyme to be a copper-containing glycoprotein.

Agaricus bisporus is a lignocellulolytic fungus, capable of degrading all the major
polymers of the plant cell wall (Wood & Leatham, 1983). Although in static liquid
culture the enzyme is freely extractable, this may be an artefact of growth in
submerged conditions. These types of fungi normally grow in moist plant residues
but not where free water is present.

Studies were initiated, therefore, to determine whether this and other
extracellular enzymes of this organism are, in fact, freely diffusible, or whether they
assume a more defined localization in closer proximity to the producing hyphal
cells. If such extracellular enzymes were localized this would give a good degree of
control over their activities; thus ensuring the efficient channelling of nutrients to
the producer organism rather than to competitors, which are present in the growth

Immunological Techniques
in Microbiology

substrate or natural environment (Wood, 1985). It is also of value to examine the sites of production of such enzymes since little published work is available to indicate in which region of the mycelium enzyme secretion occurs and if it occurs from all cells or only from specialist cells. This type of knowledge has applications both in the understanding of the role of this enzyme in the life cycle of *A. bisporus* and for the development of biotechnological approaches to the conversion of waste plant residues. Additionally, basidiomycete fungi are major pathogens of trees, and are also often responsible for biodeterioration of timber. Knowledge of the cellular localization and sites of production of enzymes responsible for biodegradation could be useful in devising methods for limiting decay of timber.

In order to locate the enzyme by electron microscopy, it has to be labelled with an electron dense marker which, in the studies reported here, is gold. Spherical colloidal gold particles, which can be prepared with consistent size (Faulk & Taylor, 1971; Horisberger, 1979; Horisberger & Tacchini-Vonlanthen, 1983) will readily adsorb various macromolecules at their surface (Hodges *et al.*, 1984). This coating, which renders the particles stable in suspension for many months without aggregation, may be used as a bridge to couple the gold to a number of different macromolecules such as lectins (Horisberger, 1981), biotins (Bonnard *et al.*, 1984), and immunoglobulins (Horisberger, 1981) which, in turn, can be used to bind specifically to the target molecule against which they are aimed. Thus the target molecule has been labelled specifically with an electron-dense marker (gold) and can be visualized in the electron microscope at high magnifications. This technique is being employed by a large number of workers on a wide range of studies. The 341 articles published in this field up to 1984 (Anon., 1984) include work in the neurosciences, endocrinology, haematology, botany, immunology and many on microbiology, although none are concerned with the fungi. As enzymes are proteins they have antigenic properties which lend themselves to the gold labelling technique described here. An antibody is raised to the fungal enzyme, the antibody is then linked to the macromolecule coating the gold and whole complex is linked to the target enzyme, thus labelling it specifically.

Materials and Methods

Culture of Agaricus bisporus

Initial experiments were designed to label laccase on the *A. bisporus* mycelial cell surface when it was grown above or within an agar substrate and to check movement of laccase within the substrate. Mycelium which had been isolated from within the pileus of a sporophore was grown on 2% malt agar at 25 °C. In order to keep the hyphae either above or below the agar surface a sterile cellophane sheet was placed on the agar with the inoculum above or below it.

Gold-label preparation

Gold particles were purchased ready prepared and coupled to a bridging antibody. For this work, as the laccase antibody was raised in a rabbit, 5 nm gold particles coupled to a goat-antirabbit antibody (GAR$_5$) were purchased from Janssen Life Sciences Products. The GAR$_5$ complex appears to be very stable and has now been stored at 4 °C for 21 months without coagulation.

Enzyme purification and antibody production

The laccase was purified (Wood, 1980a) and antiserum was prepared in a rabbit injected intramuscularly with the enzyme emulsified with Freunds Complete Adjuvant.

Applying the gold label

Pieces of cellophane bearing the aerial mycelium were cut into 2 mm squares, and the agar containing submerged mycelium into 1 mm cubes. These specimens were then submerged in laccase antibody either undiluted or diluted 1:1 with phosphate buffered saline $+0.05\%$ Tween 20 (PBS-Tween) (Clark & Adams, 1977) for 3 h at room temperature; they were then washed in 4×10 min changes of PBS-Tween followed by incubation in GAR$_5$ either undiluted, or diluted 1:10 or 1:500 with PBS-Tween, for 1 h and washed again as before.

Fixation and embedding

After gold labelling, the tissue was fixed in 2.5% glutaraldehyde in 0.2 M sodium cacodylate buffer pH 7.2 for 4 h at room temperature. The fixative was removed by 4×30 min washes in cacodylate buffer. Dehydration and embedding followed one of two methods.

Room temperature method

The tissue was passaged through an ethanol series of 25%, 50%, 70%, 80%, 90% (20 min in each) to absolute ethanol at room temperature, it was then thoroughly impregnated with Spurrs resin (Spurr, 1969) by passing through the following dilution series of resin in absolute ethanol—25%, 50%, 75%, for 24 h each and 100% resin for 48 h. The tissue pieces were then placed in fresh resin in embedding moulds and polymerized overnight at 70 °C in a fume cupboard.

Low temperature method

The tissue was passaged through the ethanol series but in this case the temperature was reduced thus: 25% at 4 °C, 50% from 4 °C to − 35 °C. It was kept at − 35 °C for the remaining dehydration steps and changes were carried out as rapidly as possible in a large insulated box of ice at $-35\,°C$. All pipettes, tubes and alcohols were kept at the same temperature. For this method, a low temperature resin (Lowicryl K_4M) was used (Carlemalm *et al.*, 1982). The resin impregnation regime was 25% resin in absolute ethanol for 1 h, 50% and 75% resin for 2 h each, 100% resin for 36 h all at $-35\,°C$. The temperature was dropped to $-40\,°C$ during the period in 100% resin.

These temperatures were maintained in a low temperature chest-type laboratory freezer with accurate temperature control.

The K_4M resin was polymerized by exposure to UV light of 360 nm and the freezer was set up for polymerization according to the resin manufacturer's recommendation as follows: The interior of the freezer was lined throughout with aluminium foil with the shiny side showing in order to obtain maximum light reflection. A UV lamp with a 15 W 37 cm Blacklight Blue F15T8/BLB tube was set up 40 cm from the specimen. The lamp holder was also covered with reflecting foil, and a foil covered baffle was placed between the lamp and the specimens to ensure that they were irradiated by reflected light only.

The resin impregnated specimens were placed in freshly made up K_4M resin in 8.0 mm diameter polythene embedding capsules, and paper labels written in Indian ink were inserted. The capsules were filled to the brim and closed with every effort being made to exclude air bubbles. The filled capsules were placed in stacking trays (Fig. 1) which were specially prepared from UV-transmitting OXO2 perspex glued with Tensol cement No 12, a dichloromethane mixture which appeared to be UV-

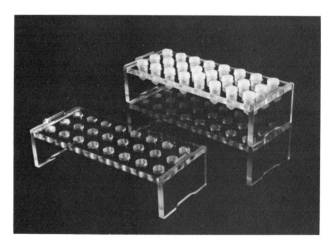

Fig. 1. Stacking trays, with and without embedding capsules, prepared from UV light transparent perspex.

transmitting. The trays were stacked in the freezer and polymerization was carried out by UV irradiation for 24 h at − 40 °C followed by 24 h at room temperature.

Sectioning and staining

Blocks were trimmed on an LKB Pyramitome with which 2 μm thick survey sections were taken and stained with azur, borax and methylene blue, all at 1% in aqueous solution in order to locate the mushroom tissue for accurate trimming. Ultra-thin sections were cut on an LKB Ultratome III ultramicrotome with a diamond knife. The sections were collected on uncoated 400 mesh copper grids and examined unstained or after staining with saturated aqueous uranyl acetate.

The steps in the treatment of specimens is summarized in the following sequential list.

1 Incubated with anti-laccase primary antibody.
2 Rinsed.
3 Incubated with goat-antirabbit antibody/gold.
4 Rinsed.
5 Fixed in glutaraldehyde.
6 Rinsed.
7 Dehydrated and embedded in resin.
8 Sectioned.
9 Examined in electron microscope.

Controls

Three controls were prepared to verify the specificity of the gold labelling.

1 The GAR_5 was applied to specimens which were not previously incubated with laccase antibody.
2 Laccase antibody was replaced with an antibody raised against White Bryony Mosaic Virus, a totally unrelated plant virus antigen.
3 No antibody or gold label was applied to the specimens which were put straight into the glutaraldehyde fixative after washing in PBS-Tween.

Results and Discussion

Specific labelling occurred at the surface of those *A. bisporus* cells which were above the agar, apparently associated with the mucilage layer surrounding the cell (Figs. 2a, b, c and 3a). The amount of label varied considerably, some cells having a continuous heavy deposit all round the periphery (Figs. 2a and b) whilst others had intermittent labelling (Fig. 2c), often denser in patches of thicker mucilage (Fig. 3a), or where it formed a bridge between adjacent cells (Fig. 3b). Many aerial cells,

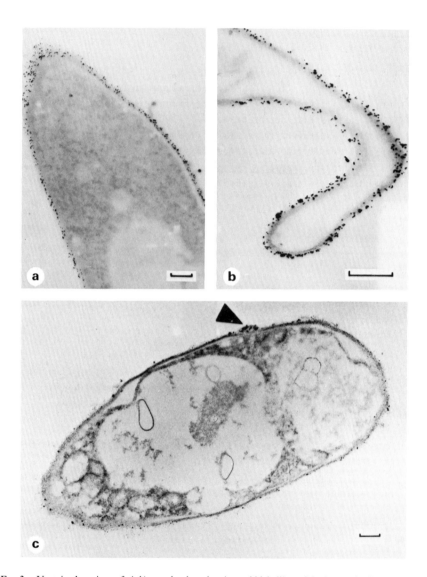

FIG. 2.   Unstained sections of *A. bisporus* hyphae showing gold labelling of the laccase in the mucilage on the cell surface. Labelling may be heavy (a & b), or light (c) but concentrated in mucilage aggregations (Arrow). Bar marks = 0.5 μm.

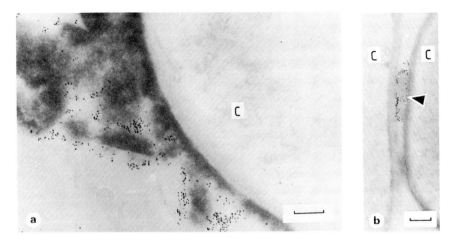

FIG. 3.   Immunogold labelled laccase in mucilage layer at cell surface (a) or arrowed (b) in mucilage 'bridge' between adjacent cells (C). Bar marks = 0.2 μm.

however, were not labelled, nor were those growing beneath the agar surface. This suggests that not all cells produce laccase and that the enzyme diffuses into the agar from submerged cells.

Control 1 had occasional gold particles at the surface (Fig. 4) but none were detected on control 2 (Fig. 5) or control 3.

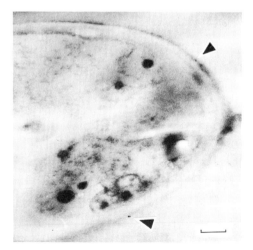

FIG. 4.   Control 1—laccase antibody omitted—showed occasional presence of gold particles (arrows). Bar mark = 0.2 μm.

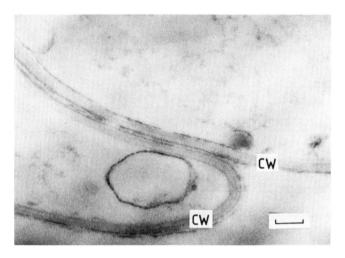

FIG. 5. Control—laccase antibody replaced with unrelated viral antibody—no gold label detected. CW = cell wall. Bar mark = 0.2 μm.

Labelling was effected with GAR_5 undiluted (Figs. 3a and b) or diluted 1:10 with PBS (Figs. 2a, b and c). None, however, was detected at a GAR_5 dilution of 1:500. The degree of labelling was the same in both Spurrs and K_4M resin. In all treatments the contrast was low, and the cell components were poorly defined, due to the omission of osmium tetroxide secondary fixation and to the fact that, to avoid obscuring the gold, heavy metal stains were not generally applied to the sections. Contrast could, however, be improved by staining with uranyl acetate without obscuring the gold particles. Apart from difficulty in identifying organelles, the main problem was that of focussing specimens of very low contrast. If the specimen is not in, or fairly near focus, the gold particles can easily become invisible or difficult to distinguish (Figs. 6a and b). When gold labelling was carried out before fixation and embedding, the label survived both the heat-polymerized Spurr's resin (Figs. 2a, b and c) and the low temperature UV light-polymerized Lowicryl K_4M resin (Figs. 3a and b). It has been suggested, however (Roth, 1984), that where labelling is to take place on the thin sections after embedding, some loss of antigenic activity may occur with heat polymerization and in such cases K_4M is recommended. Studies are in progress to evaluate this in relation to laccase and *A. bisporus*. Lowicryl apparently did not penetrate the fungal cells sufficiently well in the infiltration times used, thus causing fragile sections with frequent holes. A longer infiltration time should overcome this problem.

A technical problem which caused considerable difficulty was the fact that when the fungal tissue was fixed without osmium tetroxide (which would blacken it) and embedded in resin, it became invisible which made block trimming and orientation

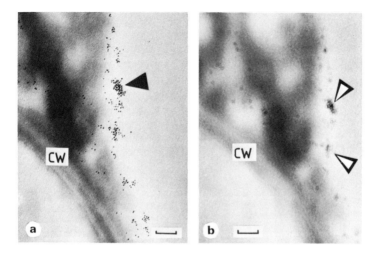

Fig. 6.   Gold label (arrows) on laccase, (a) electron microscope in focus. (b) Same area with the microscope slightly out of focus. If the microscope is farther from focus the gold particles can be overlooked. CW = cell wall. Bar marks = 0.2 μm.

very difficult. Furthermore, where the mycelial colony was above and below the agar, the agar was also rendered invisible so that it was impossible to determine the position of the mycelium. These problems were largely overcome in two ways: firstly, the blue stained survey section for light microscopy usually revealed the mycelial cells, although they were often in very low numbers; secondly, the use of a cellophane sheet on the agar surface enabled the aerial hyphae to be separated from the submerged hyphae. When treating the aerial hyphae prior to embedding, handling was somewhat difficult as the tissue tended to separate from the cellophane and roll up into a ball. This could be partially overcome during the initial cutting of the tissue pieces which should be cut on the cellophane backing using a very sharp round-bladed scalpel such as a Swann Morton 22. The cut should be made by rolling the blade as the normal slicing cut will drag the mycelium from the cellophane.

To ensure that specific labelling is being achieved it is vital that adequate controls are used, that the antiserum titre and affinity is well understood, and that the effects of dilutions of the antibody and the gold label are fully investigated.

This work is being continued in attempt to locate the sites of laccase activity on the substrate and its distribution within the *A. bisporus* cell.

Conclusion

The results described here have indicated that this technique enables fungal enzymes to be visualized and detected with high resolution. It should thus be possible to determine very accurately the location of a range of fungal enzymes within and on the surface of fungi and in their growth substrates; provided that such enzymes can be extracted, purified and used to produce good antibodies. The applications should be far reaching, not only in the study of the cultivated mushroom and its relationship with the compost upon which it grows, but also to the wood rotting fungi, and in the study of hyperparasitic fungal activity which is receiving so much interest in the field of biological control of plant diseases.

Great care must, however, always be given to the preparation of adequate controls if confidence is to be maintained in the specificity of the labelling.

Acknowledgements

We would like to thank Mr S. Coggins for making the embedding racks and Mr S. Matcham and Mr J. Pegler for technical assistance.

References

ANON. 1984 *Colloidal Metal Marking Reference Book* Vols 1 and 2. Beerse, Belgium: Jannsen Life Science Products.

BONNARD, C., PAPERMASTER, D. S. & KRAEHENBUHL, J-P. 1984 The streptavidin–biotin bridge technique: application in light and electron microscope immunocytochemistry. In *Immunolabelling for Electron Microscopy* eds. Polak, J. M. & Varndell, I. M. pp. 95–111. Amsterdam: Elsevier Science Publishers BV.

CARLEMALM, E., GARAVITO, M. & VILLIGER, W. 1982 Resin development for electron microscopy and an analysis of embedding at low temperature. *Journal of Microscopy* 126, 123–143.

CLARK, M. F. & ADAMS, A. N. 1977 Characteristics of the microplate method of enzyme-linked immunosorbent assay (ELISA) for the detection of plant viruses. *Journal of General Virology* 34, 475–483.

FAULK, W. P. & TAYLOR, G. M. 1971 An immunocolloid method for the electron microscope. *Immunochemistry* 8, 1081–1083.

HODGES, G. M., SMOLIRA, M. A. & LIVINGSTON, D. C. 1984 Scanning electron microscope immunocytochemistry in practice. In *Immunolabelling for Electron Microscopy* eds. Polak, J. M. & Varndell, I. M. pp. 189–233. Amsterdam: Elsevier Science Publishers BV.

HORISBERGER, M. 1979 Evaluation of colloidal gold as a cytochemical marker for transmission and scanning electron microscopy. *Biologie Cellulaire* 36, 253–258.

HORISBERGER, M. 1981 Colloidal gold: a cytochemical marker for light and fluorescent microscopy and for transmission and scanning electron microscopy. In *Scanning Electron Microscopy Vol. II* ed. Johari, O. pp. 9–28. Chicago: SEM Inc. AMF O'Hare.

HORISBERGER, M. & TACCHINI-VONLANTHEN, M. 1983 Ultrastructural localization of Kunitz inhibitor on thin sections of *Glycine max* (Soybean) cv. Maple Arrow by the gold method. *Histochemistry* 77, 37–50.

ROTH, J. 1984 The protein A-gold technique for antigen localisation in tissue sections by light and electron microscopy. In *Immunolabelling for Electron Microscopy* eds. Polak, J. M. and Varndell, I. M. pp. 113–121. Amsterdam: Elsevier Science Publishers BV.

Spurr, A. R. 1969 A low viscosity epoxy resin embedding medium for electron microscopy. *Journal of Ultrastructure Research* **26**, 31–43.

Wood, D. A. 1979 A method of estimating biomass of *Agaricus bisporus* in a solid substrate, composted wheat straw. *Biotechnology Letters* **1**, 255–260.

Wood, D. A. 1980a Production, purification and properties of laccase of *Agaricus bisporus*. *Journal of General Microbiology* **117**, 327–338.

Wood, D. A. 1980b Inactivation of extracellular laccase during fruiting of *Agaricus bisporus*. *Journal of General Microbiology* **117**, 339–345.

Wood, D. A. 1984 Microbial processes in mushroom cultivation: A large scale solid substrate fermentation. *Journal of Chemical Technology and Biotechnology* **34B**, 232–240.

Wood, D. A. 1985 Production and rates of extracellular enzymes during morphogenesis of basidiomycete fungi. In *Developmental Biology of Higher Fungi* eds. Moore, D., Casseton, L. A., Wood, D. A. & Frankland, J. C. pp. 375–387. Cambridge: Cambridge University Press.

Wood, D. A. & Goodenough, P. 1977 Fruiting of *Agaricus bisporus*: changes in extracellular enzyme activity during growth and fruiting. *Archives of Microbiology* **114**, 161–165.

Wood, D. A. & Leatham, G. F. 1983 Lignocellulose degradation during the life cycle of *Agaricus bisporus*. Federation of European Microbiological Societies. *Microbiology Letters* **20**, 421–424.

Immunofluorescent Techniques for Legionnaires' Disease

M. G. SMITH

Microbiology Department, Kingston Hospital, Galsworthy Road, Kingston Upon Thames, Surrey KT2 7BG

Introduction

The indirect immunofluorescent or 'sandwich' technique is a simple technique involving the attachment of an antibody to an antigen and, after washing, the attachment of a fluorescein isothiocyanate (FITC) conjugated antiglobulin to the first antibody which renders the antigen visible when viewed under a microscope set up for fluorescence.

Indirect immunofluorescence may be applied to the diagnosis of Legionnaires' Disease in two different ways, the detection of antibodies to *Legionella pneumophila* in the patient's serum and the detection of *Legionella* organisms in specimens from the respiratory tract.

The use of the formolized yolk-sac antigen has been shown to eliminate false positives in the antibody test (Taylor *et al.*, 1979) and has been adopted by the Public Health Laboratory Service as one of the standard techniques available for the diagnosis of *L. pneumophila* infections. Any laboratory having access to a suitable microscope will, by using the method described later, be able to add this investigation to their set of routine tests.

The time for seroconversion in patients infected with *L. pneumophila* can vary from 1 week to 6 weeks or more (Edelstein *et al.*, 1980), thus making the antibody test less suitable for rapid diagnosis in acute infections. Detection of the organism in the early stages of the disease can be of great help to clinicians and may be attempted on a variety of specimens obtained from the respiratory tract, although lung biopsies and secretions obtained by bronchoscopy are preferable to expectorated sputum. Direct immunofluorescence is a widely used technique (Cherry & McKinney, 1979), but it requires the availability of FITC-conjugated antisera. The indirect immunofluorescent technique described in this chapter is more convenient in that any number of unconjugated *Legionella* specific antisera may be used with a single FITC-conjugated antiglobulin.

Immunological Techniques
in Microbiology

Any immunological technique used to detect the presence of an organism is limited to the range of antisera available and it is therefore advisable that attempts should be made to isolate the organism by means of cultivation from any specimen received. This is the means by which infections by new serogroups or species of *Legionella* can be discovered.

Materials and Methods

Serum antibody detection

Materials required

Phosphate buffered saline pH 7.2 (PBS); PTFE-coated multi-test slides with 3 mm wells (Flow Laboratories); Formalin-killed yolk-sac antigen (FYSA) of *Legionella pneumophila* serogroup 1 (Division of Microbiological Reagents and Quality Control (DMRQC), Central Public Health Laboratory); FITC conjugated anti-human globulin (Wellcome Diagnostics); Buffered Glycerol Mounting Medium pH 9 (Difco Laboratories).

Procedure

1 Pipette 5 µl volumes of FYSA onto each well of a multi-test slide and allow to dry in a 37 °C incubator. Fix the antigen by placing the slide in acetone at room temperature for 15 min.

2 Make doubling dilutions of the serum under test in PBS from 1/16 to 1/2048. (If large numbers of sera are to be tested they may be screened at a dilution of 1/16.) Add 10 µl volumes to the antigen wells and incubate the slides at 37 °C for 30 min in a humidity box. Positive (DMRQC) and negative control sera must be included with each batch of tests.

3 Rinse the slides with PBS and then wash with gentle agitation for 15 min in a glass staining jar with two changes of PBS. Rinse the slides in distilled water and allow to dry at 37 °C.

4 Dilute the anti-human conjugate to its in-use dilution (determined by 'chessboard' titrations against a standard serum). Add 5 µl to each antigen well and incubate the slides at 37 °C for 30 min as before.

5 .Repeat step 3.

6 Mount the slides in buffered glycerol and examine under a microscope using incident fluorescence with a magnification of around 500 × with filtration set for FITC. A suitable system is a Leitz microscope with 50 W mercury vapour light source, filter block I2, 50 × water immersion objective and 10 × eye pieces.

7 The intensity of fluorescence of the individual bacilli is scored $+++$, $++$, $+$, $\pm$ and $-$. The end point is the last dilution to show $+$ fluorescence. The

positive control serum should show + fluorescence at its stated end point. The negative control should show no fluorescence.

Interpretation

Where paired sera are tested, a fourfold rise in titre to at least 64 is diagnostic of an infection with *L. pneumophila*. A single serum with a titre $\geqslant 256$ and a relevant clinical history is also accepted as being diagnostic.

If sera have only been screened at a dilution of 1/16 then any that show + fluorescence must be titrated to determine the end point.

Sera with a titre $\geqslant 16$ should be referred to a specialist laboratory for further study using antigens of the other serogroups of *L. pneumophila*. Low titres with serogroup 1 antigen may indicate infection with other serogroups.

Comments

Reconstituted but undiluted conjugates should be stored in aliquots at $-20\,°C$, diluted conjugates may be stored at $4\,°C$ and used for up to 1 week. Positive control sera should be diluted 1/16 in PBS and stored in aliquots at $-20\,°C$.

Detection of L. pneumophila *in fresh clinical specimens and formalin fixed post-mortem samples*

Materials required

PBS pH 7.2; PBS containing 10% formalin (formol PBS); PTFE-coated multi-test slides with 6 mm wells (Flow Laboratories); plain microscope slides; polyvalent rabbit antiserum to *L. pneumophila* serogroups 1 to 6 (DMRQC); normal rabbit serum; FITC conjugated antirabbit gamma-globulin (Behring); Buffered Glycerol Mounting Medium pH 9 (Difco).

Slide preparation from fresh specimens (sputum, aspirations, biopsies, etc.)

1 Make 15 mm diameter smears of the specimen on two plain microscope slides and allow to dry in a 37 °C incubator. Label them as test and control. Gently heat-fix the smears in a Bunsen flame.
2 Place the slides in a humidity box and cover the smears with formol PBS. After 20 min at room temperature gently rinse the slides in distilled water and allow to dry as before. Include a known positive specimen if available.

Slide preparation from formalin-fixed specimens (lung)

1 Make a cut through a consolidated portion of the specimen using a scalpel, blot the cut surface on paper tissue and scrape the cut surface with the scalpel. Re-suspend the scrapings in 0.1 ml of PBS.

2 Pipette 5 µl of the suspension onto duplicate wells on each of two multi–test slides and allow to dry in a 37 °C incubator. Label the slides as test and control. Gently heat fix the slides in a Bunsen flame. Include a known positive specimen if available.

Procedure

1 Make a 1/100 dilution of the polyvalent antiserum and normal rabbit serum in PBS.

2 Cover the test smears/wells with the polyvalent serum and cover the control smears/wells with the normal rabbit serum. Incubate for 30 min at 37 °C in a humidity box.

3 Rinse the slides in PBS and then wash with gentle agitation for 15 min in a glass staining jar with two changes of PBS. Rinse the slides in distilled water and allow to dry at 37 °C.

4 Dilute the antirabbit conjugate to its in–use dilution (determined by 'chessboard' titrations against a standard serum and antigen). Cover test and control smears/wells with the conjugate and incubate the slides at 37 °C for 30 min as before.

5 Repeat step 3.

6 Mount the slides in buffered glycerol and examine under a microscope using incident fluorescence with a magnification of around 500 × with filtration set for FITC.

7 *L. pneumophila* stain as fluorescent pleomorphic cocco–bacilli.

Interpretation

The presence of 25 or more strongly fluorescent bacilli only in the test smear/well should be reported as positive. Care, however, must be exercised when examining sputum, trans–tracheal aspirations and specimens obtained by bronchoscopy due to the presence of other bacteria which may fluoresce with the natural antibodies present in rabbit serum. In addition, some strains of *Pseudomonas fluorescens* fluoresce with the specific *Legionella* antiserum although their morphology may be sufficiently different to prevent them being mistaken for *L. pneumophila*.

Comments

As samples of tissue containing *L. pneumophila* for use as positive controls are not always available, the FYSA used for detecting serum antibodies may be used as a suitable substitute.

The polyvalent antiserum should be diluted 1/10 in PBS and stored in aliquots at − 20 °C. The reconstituted but undiluted conjugate should be stored in aliquots at − 20 °C. In–use dilutions of both may be stored at 4 °C and used for up to 1 week.

The methods described here are based on those recommended by the DMRQC, Director A. G. Taylor.

References

CHERRY, W. B. & McKINNEY, R. M. 1979 Detection of Legionnaires' Disease Bacteria. In *Clinical Specimens by Direct Immunofluorescence in "Legionnaires'"*: *The Disease, The Bacterium & Methodology* ed. Jones, G. L. & Hebert, G. A. pp. 92–98. Atlanta: U.S. Department of Health, Education and Welfare, Center for Disease Control.

EDELSTEIN, P. H., MEYER, R. D. & FINEGOLD, S. M. 1980 Laboratory diagnosis of Legionnaires' disease, *American Review of Respiratory Disease* 21, 317–327.

TAYLOR, A. G., HARRISON, T. G., DIGHERO, M. W. & BRADSTREET, C. M. P. 1979 False positive reactions in the indirect fluorescent antibody test for Legionnaires' disease eliminated by use of formalised yolk-sac antigen. *Annals of Internal Medicine* 90, 686–689.

Immunofluorescence Techniques in Plant Pathology

D. E. STEAD

Ministry of Agriculture, Fisheries and Food, Harpenden Laboratory, Hatching Green, Harpenden, Herts AL5 2BD

Introduction

Immunofluorescence (IF) techniques are particularly useful in the diagnosis of many bacterial plant diseases. They may be used to identify bacterial cultures isolated from diseased tissues but they are more frequently used to detect the presence of pathogens in diseased or latently infected plant tissues. They are particularly useful for the detection of pathogens in seed and other propagating organs, e.g. potato tubers. In this context they are often considered to be more useful than other serodetection or diagnostic methods such as enzyme linked immunosorbent assays (ELISA) or latex agglutination, because the serological reaction is visualized on the cell surface. This usually allows differentiation of the target bacterium from cross-reacting bacteria and non-specific reactions which show weak, patchy or incomplete fluorescence.

In the simplest methods, the suspected target bacteria or bacterial fractions of comminuted plant tissues are suspended in a suitable buffer and samples are pipetted onto the surface of clean glass microscope slides. After air drying and fixing using heat, ethanol or formalin the smear is covered with antiserum. In direct immunofluorescence tests the antibodies are conjugated to a fluorescent substance, usually fluorescein isothiocyanate (FITC) or occasionally tetramethylrhodamine isothiocyanate (TRITC). In indirect tests an additional step is included. The fixed antigen is incubated with the antiserum (produced, for example, in rabbit). After washing, a second antiserum produced against rabbit immunoglobulin, usually in sheep or goat and conjugated to FITC, is added. After washing, the smears are mounted in glycerol, buffered at high pH to enhance fluorescence, before observing with a microscope fitted with epifluorescent illumination and filters suitable for use with FITC or TRITC. Cells are visualized as a peripheral ring of fluorescence against a dark background.

For this type of application, indirect methods are often considered more useful. They have the advantages of amplification of the fluorescence and, provided all

Immunological Techniques
in Microbiology

0–632–01908–5

antisera to bacteria are produced in the same animal species (usually rabbit), a single commercially available FITC conjugate can be used for all diseases. Direct methods, however, often have greater specificity.

Methods for labelling antisera with fluorescein are described by Chantler (1982) and Goldman (1968) and equipment required for IF tests is described by Heimer (1982). For principles of immunofluorescence see Nairn (1976), Goldman (1968) and Johnson *et al.* (1978).

The methods given are for a simple indirect IF test. When bacteria cannot be readily separated from plant debris or when autofluorescing substances interfere with the test, immunosorbent immunofluorescence (ISIF) may be used. The microscope slide is coated with antibodies and after incubation with the test suspension, plant debris or other bacteria are washed off leaving the target bacteria fixed to the slide (Van Vuurde *et al.*, 1983; Van Vuurde & Van Henten, 1983; Van Vuurde, 1987). Cells are visualized by a direct IF test and for this, FITC conjugates must be prepared (Chantler, 1982).

Materials and Methods

Microscope

The microscope should be fitted with an epifluorescent lamp preferably high pressure mercury vapour or high pressure xenon, for example HBO 50 W or XBO 150 W. These produce light of the correct wavelengths to excite fluorescein. A set of filters is required that will further remove unnecessary wavelengths and also remove wavelengths of fluorescent emission that would otherwise swamp the image.

Epifluorescence uses the objective lens as condenser and so it may be useful to have an objective lens with an integral iris diaphragm. Objectives with lowest possible magnification and highest possible numerical aperture are best. An X63 oil immersion planapochromatic lens is particularly useful but X40 dry objectives are also useful.

Slides

PTFE coated multi-spot slides (10 and 12 windows) are commercially available. Otherwise circles (1 cm diameter) can be inscribed with a diamond on clean glass slides. Slides are cleaned in ethanol before use.

Antisera

The author produces most antisera to live whole cell preparations in rabbits, by a course of either intramuscular or intravenous injections. For whole cells, specificity appears to be greatest with short series of intravenous injections but for some groups of bacteria, a series of several weekly intramuscular injections, after emulsification with Freund's Incomplete Adjuvant, gives higher titres.

Titres (reciprocal of highest dilution giving optimum fluorescence) are determined by indirect IF tests. Antisera are usually semi-purified by ammonium sulphate precipitation and the titres are re-determined. Antisera with titres > 1:500 are usually suitable for IF tests. An antiserum working dilution, usually half the dilution at titre, can be selected but it is preferable to work with short series of antiserum dilutions just below the titre. Cross reactions with closely related bacteria may occur at low antiserum dilutions (1:10–1:40). At greater dilutions, fluorescence may still occur but will usually be patchy, weak, or incomplete. Antisera are diluted in either 0.01 M phosphate buffer pH 7.2 or quarter strength Ringers solution containing Tween 20 and peptone (RTP) where blocking with protein is required. In ISIF antibodies are coated to suitable solid phases using carbonate coating buffer pH 9.6. Blocking with protein and the use of detergent may significantly increase specificity and reduce background staining. They are particularly important in immunosorbent IF.

Antigens

All tests should contain a positive control with the target bacterium for comparative purposes. When possible, use 24–48 hour-old, well-isolated colonies with typical colony characteristics. When used at a single dilution, suspend cells at a population of approximately 5×10^5 cells/ml of 0.05 M phosphate buffer pH 7.0. Inclusion of 0.05% Tween 20 may prevent cell clumping during drying. When attempting to detect bacteria in plant tissues, the use of known diseased material as an extra control is advised. Comminute plant tissues and prepare dilutions series (usually neat, 1:10, 1:100 and 1:1000) in 0.05 M phosphate buffer pH 7.0. In all tests it is preferable to include a dilution series of antiserum and antigen to avoid problems of antibody or antigen excess.

FITC conjugates

These can be prepared by the methods of Chantler (1982) and for direct IF tests this is usually necessary. For indirect IF tests with antisera produced in rabbits, sheep or goat antirabbit immunoglobulin conjugated to FITC can be purchased from the Sigma Chemical Company or Wellcome Laboratories. The working dilution is determined by carrying out a chequerboard titration of antibody and FITC conjugate dilutions. For most commercial preparations, the optimum working dilution is between 1:50 and 1:500. The working dilution is the highest at which good fluorescence occurs. Conjugates should be used at this dilution to minimise background staining or non-specific attachment to cells (often seen as 'ghosts').

Buffers

1 0.05 M phosphate buffer   pH 7.0
   Na_2HPO_4 4.26 g
   KH_2PO_4 2.72 g
   distilled water   1 litre
2. 0.01 M phosphate buffer   pH 7.2
   $Na_2HPO_4.12H_2O$ 2.7 g
   $NaH_2PO_4.2H_2O$ 0.4 g
   distilled water   1 litre
3 0.1 M phosphate buffered glycerine   pH 7.6
   $Na_2HPO_4.12H_2O$ 3.2 g
   NaH_2PO_4 0.15 g
   glycerine   50 ml
   distilled water   100 ml
4 Quarter strength Ringers Tween Peptone Buffer (RTP)
   NaCl   1.75 g
   KCl   0.1 g
   $CaCl_2$ 0.12 g
   $NaHCO_3$ 0.05 g
   Tween 20   0.05 ml
   peptone   1.0 g
   distilled water   1 litre
5 Carbonate coating buffer
   Na_2CO_3 1.5 g
   $NaHCO_3$ 2.93 g
   distilled water   1 litre

Basic procedure for indirect IF

1 Add bacterial suspension at appropriate dilution in 0.05 M phosphate buffer pH 7.0 to all windows on the slide (25 μl for a 6 mm diameter window). Allow to air dry in a laminar airflow cabinet or at 37 °C. If this results in uneven drying and subsequent clumping, use a smaller volume or else spread the volume within a 1 cm circle inscribed with a diamond on a clean microscope slide, or repeat using buffer containing 0.05% (v/v) Tween 20. Prepare slides with a pure suspension of known bacterium to which antiserum was made and also with comminuted tissue showing typical symptoms, if available.

2 Fix by gently heating in a Bunsen flame (as for Gram stain) or in 3% formalin in phosphate buffer for 10 min followed by a 5 min wash in buffer.

3 Add sufficient antiserum at appropriate dilution to cover the window. Cover one window with pre-immune serum at the antiserum working dilution. Cover at least one window with buffer instead of antiserum (FITC conjugate control). Incubate for 30 min in a humid chamber at room temperature.

4 Rinse off antisera and wash for 3 min in each of three changes of 0.01 M phosphate buffer (pH 7.2) in a Coplin jar. Keep positive control slides in a separate jar to avoid cross contamination.

5 Take up excess moisture with absorbent paper avoiding cross contamination between windows. Blotting dry may remove preparations.

6 Add sufficient FITC conjugate at the working dilution to cover each window. Incubate for 30 min in a dark humid chamber at room temperature.

7 Rinse and wash as in **4**.

8 Take up excess moisture.

9 Add 5–10 μl of phosphate buffered glycerine pH 7.6. Cover with a large coverslip and observe. Scan two window diameters at right angles and approximately one radian along the edge of the window. Observe for bright green peripheral fluorescence of cells. Read control windows first. If fluorescent cells are observed in the pre-immune serum and FITC conjugate control windows, repeat the procedure. If fluorescent cells are still found, discard the slides and use a different antiserum or FITC conjugate preparation.

Immunosorbent IF procedure (based upon the methods of Van Vuurde *et al.*, 1983 and Van Vuurde & Van Henton, 1983)

1 To each window pipette a small droplet of commercial nail varnish dissolved in acetone (33% v/v). Take up the excess and air dry the slide.

2 Cover the window with antiserum diluted 1:100 v/v in carbonate coating buffer pH 9.6. Leave at least one window blank. Incubate overnight at 4 °C or for 30 min at 25 °C.

3 Wash twice (5 min each) with quarter strength Ringer's solution containing 0.05% v/v Tween 20 and 0.1% w/v peptone (RTP).

4 Allow to air dry.

5 Cover the windows with the bacterial suspension at several dilutions (usually neat, 1:10, 1:100, 1:1000). Incubate at 25 °C for 1 h.

6 Wash in RTP and take up excess liquid.

7 Cover all windows with the FITC-antibody conjugate at appropriate dilutions in a short series just below the titre. Incubate for 30 min at 25 °C.

8 Rinse and wash in RTP and take up excess liquid.

9 Add 5–10 μl phosphate buffered glycerine pH 7.6 and observe as for the indirect IF procedure.

Results

The indirect IF method given has been used successfully for the identification of several plant pathogenic bacteria isolated in pure culture from diseased plant

TABLE 1. *Applications of immunofluorescent techniques for bacterial diseases of plants*

Bacterium	Disease	Identifi-cation	Detection of bacterium	
			Diseased tissue	Latent/seed infection
Clavibacter michiganense subsp. *michiganense*	Bacterial canker of tomato	+	+	+
Clavibacter michiganense subsp. *sepedonicum*	Ring rot of potatoes	+	+	+
Clavibacter michiganense subsp. *insidiosum*	Wilt of lucerne	+	nd	nd
Erwinia amylovora	Fireblight of rosaceous hosts	+	+	+
Erwinia carotovora subsp. *atroseptica*	Blackleg of potatoes	I	+	+
Erwinia carotovora subsp. *carotovora*	Soft rot of potatoes and other hosts	+	+	+
Erwinia chrysanthemi	Soft rot/wilt of many hosts	+	nd	nd
Pseudomonas syringae pv. *pisi*	Bacterial blight of peas	+	+	+
Pseudomonas solanacearum	Brown rot of potatoes	+	+	nd

nd = not done.

material. The technique has also been used to detect the presence of the many bacterial pathogens in diseased and latently infected plant tissues. Table 1 lists these applications.

Discussion

Several other applications of IF techniques have been reported. Several reports discuss the problems encountered in development of the tests (Trigalet *et al.*, 1978; Crowley & De Boer, 1982; Stead *et al.*, 1987). Most of the major groups of plant pathogenic bacteria are represented. They include methods for detection of pathogens in seeds (Coleno, 1968; Schaad, 1978; Schaad & Donaldson, 1980; Malin *et al.*, 1983; Van Vuurde *et al.*, 1983); methods for detection of pathogens in seed potatoes (Allen & Kelman, 1977; Vruggink & De Boer, 1978; De Boer & Copeman, 1980; Crowley & De Boer, 1982; Miller, 1984; Stead *et al.*, 1987) and methods for detection of infections in trees (Miller, 1983).

Immunofluorescence techniques are particularly useful for the detection and diagnosis of plant pathogenic bacteria but there are several possible limiting factors.

When many other bacteria are present cross-reactions and non-specific staining may occur. The methods given attempt to reduce the possibility of these reactions occurring by using detergents such as Tween 20 and blocking agents such as peptone but it may be necessary to include other controls. Background staining may be reduced by counterstaining with, for example, Evans Blue (Goldman, 1968). Background staining may be a problem if the fluorochrome: protein ratio (F:P) is high, e.g. > 4. Many commercially available preparations give this ratio but, if not available, it should be calculated. This is especially important if you prepare your own FITC conjugates. For further details see Goldman (1968) and Chantler (1982).

Antisera prepared against whole cells will contain antibodies against soluble and insoluble antigens. Suspension of bacteria in buffers will release some of the soluble antigens. Unless washed off, these will coat the slide as it dries and this may contribute to background staining. Careful washing of cell suspensions and of fixed smears may reduce this staining. Attention should perhaps be given to the culture medium. High sugar content may favour increased production of soluble extracellular polysaccharides, which are antigenic.

When it is difficult to remove plant debris from the test suspension, the efficacy of IF may be impaired. For example, tissue containing bacteria may be lost from the slide during washing. The presence of plant particles will create a three-dimensional layer in which it may be difficult to see fluorescing cells. Immunosorbent IF is one possible means of overcoming this problem but it should be borne in mind that the bacteria must come into contact with the antibody layer and must remain adsorbed to it during the remainder of the test. The properties of antibodies differ even within the same class and one antibody preparation that is useful in IF may not be useful as the trapping layer in ISIF. The antibody concentration on the solid phase may be critical. The possibility of other bacteria or the FITC conjugate adsorbing non-specifically to the solid phase should not be overlooked. The development of any immunosorbent IF testing procedure must take into account most of these and perhaps other factors.

References

ALLEN, E. & KELMAN, A. 1977 Immunofluorescent stain procedures for detection and identification of *Erwinia carotovora* var. *atroseptica*. *Phytopathology* 67, 1305–1312.

CHANTLER, S. M. 1982 Labelling antisera with fluorescein. *Immunofluorescence techniques in diagnostic microbiology*. Public Health Laboratory Service Monograph Series No. 18 eds. Edwards, J. M. B., Taylor, C. E. D. & Tomlinson, A. H. pp. 14–19. London: HMSO.

COLENO, A. 1968 Utilisation de la technique d'immunofluorescence pour le depistage de *Pseudomonas phaseolicola* (Burkh.) Dowson dans les lots de semences contaminees. *Comptes Rendus de l'Academie d'Agriculture Francaise* 54, 1016–1020.

CROWLEY, C. F. & DE BOER, S. H. 1982 Non-pathogenic bacteria associated with *Corynebacterium sepedonicum* antisera in immunofluorescence. *American Potato Journal* 59, 1–8.

DE BOER, S. J. & COPEMAN, R. J. 1980 Bacterial Ring Rot testing with the indirect fluorescent antibody staining procedure. *American Potato Journal* 57, 457–465.

GOLDMAN, M. 1968 *Fluorescent Antibody Methods*. New York: Academic Press.

HEIMER, G. V. 1982 Fluorescence microscopy. In *Immunofluorescence Techniques in Diagnostic Microbiology*. Public Health Laboratory Service Monograph Series No. 18 eds. Edwards, J. M. B., Taylor, C. E. D. & Tomlinson, A. H., pp. 1–13. London: HMSO.

JOHNSON, G. D., HOLBORROW, E. J. & DORLING, J. 1978 Immunofluorescence and immunoenzyme techniques. In *Handbook of Experimental Immunology*, 3rd Edn. Vol. 1 ed. Weir, D. M. pp. 15.1–15.30. Oxford: Blackwell Scientific Publications.

MALIN, E. M., ROTH, D. A. & BELDEN, E. L. 1983 Indirect immunofluorescent staining for detection and identification of *Xanthomonas campestris* pv. *phaseoli* in naturally infected bean seed. *Plant Disease* 67, 645–647.

MILLER, H. J. 1983 Some factors influencing immunofluorescence microscopy as applied in diagnostic phytobacteriology with regard to *Erwinia amylovora*. *Phytopathologisches Zeitung* 108, 235–241.

MILLER, H. J. 1984 A method for the detection of latent ringrot in potatoes by immunofluorescence microscopy. *Potato Research* 27, 33–42.

NAIRN, R. C. 1976 *Fluorescent Protein Tracing*, 4th Edn. Edinburgh: Churchill Livingstone.

SCHAAD, N. W. 1978 Use of direct and indirect immunofluorescence tests for identification of *Xanthomonas campestris*. *Phytopathology* 68, 249–252.

SCHAAD, N. W. & DONALDSON, R. C. 1980 Comparison of two methods for detection of *Xanthomonas cámpestris* in infected crucifer seeds. *Seed Science and Technology* 8, 383–391.

STEAD, D. E., SELLWOOD, J. E. & RICHMOND, T. 1987 Problems with the detection of latent infections of bacterial ring rot in potato tubers by indirect fluorescent antibody tests. In *Proceedings of the 6th International Conference on Plant Pathology and Bacteriology*, Beltsville, U.S.A.: Nijhoff-Junk (In press).

TRIGALET, A., SAMSON, R. & COLENO, A. 1978 Problems related to the use of serology in phytobacteriology. In *Proceedings of the 4th International Conference on Plant Pathology and Bacteriology*, 895–902. Angers, France: INRA.

VAN VUURDE, J. W. L. 1987 Detecting seed borne bacteria by immuno-fluorescence. In *Proceedings of the 6th International Conference on Plant Pathology and Bacteriology*, Beltsville, U.S.A.: Nijhoff-Junk (In press).

VAN VUURDE, J. W. L., VAN DEN BOVENKAMP, G. W. & BIRNBAUM, Y. 1983 Immunofluorescence microscopy and enzyme-linked immunosorbent assay as potential routine tests for the detection of *Pseudomonas syringae* pv. *phaseolicola* and *Xanthomonas campestris* pv. *phaseoli* in bean seed. *Seed Science and Technology* 11, 547–559.

VAN VUURDE, J. W. L. & VAN HENTEN, C. 1983 Immunosorbent immunofluorescence microscopy (ISIF) and immunosorbent dilution plating (ISDP): New methods for the detection of plant pathogenic bacteria. *Seed Science and Technology* 11, 523–533.

VRUGGINK, H. & DE BOER, S. H. 1978 Detection of *Erwinia carotovora* var. *atroseptica* in potato tubers with immunofluorescence following induction of decay. *Potato Research* 21, 225–229.

Counter-Current Immunoelectrophoresis for the Rapid Detection of Bacterial Polysaccharide Antigen in Body Fluids

MICHELE F. MCINTYRE

Public Health Laboratory, Dulwich Hospital, East Dulwich Grove, London SE22 8QF

Introduction

Rapid techniques for the diagnosis of infections by detection of bacterial (or other microbial) antigens are relevant to patient care because: (1) isolation of a microbial pathogen may be difficult or impossible if the patient has already been treated or partially treated with an anti-microbial agent or agents, even inappropriate ones. (2) Isolation of a microbial pathogen in pure culture may be relatively slow. (3) A rapid diagnostic technique may permit the prescription of prompt 'best-guess' anti-microbial therapy.

History

Counter-current immunoelectrophoresis (CIE) was first used by Bussard (1959) to demonstrate specific meningococcal polysaccharides in cerebrospinal fluid (CSF) and serum. The technique was modified by Prince & Burke (1970) to detect Australia antigen and by Greenwood *et al.* (1971) to show the presence of specific meningococcal polysaccharides in CSF and serum. It was used in this laboratory for the detection of pneumococcal antigen by El Refaie & Dulake (1975) and *Haemophilus influenzae* antigen by McIntyre (1978).

Principle

CIE is an immunoprecipitation reaction based on immunodiffusion which is accelerated by electrophoresis. Electrophoresis also deters the radial diffusion which occurs in the Outcherlony double immunodiffusion technique.

In the CIE system, paired wells are cut in agarose layered on a glass slide. The

Immunological Techniques
in Microbiology

specimen to be tested for the presence of antigen is placed in one well of a pair and the antiserum containing antibody specific for the suspected antigen is placed in the opposite well. An electric current is passed across the agarose. Bacterial polysaccharide antigens are negatively charged and migrate towards the anode. The test specimen is placed in the cathodic well. Antisera containing specific antibodies are placed in the anodic wells and move towards the cathode by endosmosis with the normal flow of buffer. This results in the formation of a precipitation line midway between the wells where there is an optimum proportion of antigen and its specific antibody.

Compared with Outcherlony double immunodiffusion the sensitivity of CIE is increased 10- to 100-fold because the antigen-antibody reaction occurs in a region where radial diffusion has been prevented by passage of the electric current which also speeds up the process.

Materials and Methods

Apparatus

The standard electrophoretic tank (Shandon Southern Instruments Ltd, U.K.) is used with a Vokam power pack (Shandon).

Veronal buffer solution for the tank

This contains (g/l): sodium 5,5-diethyl barbiturate, 10.31; 5,5-diethyl barbituric acid, 0.92; sodium acetate, 6.80; pH 8.6. No preservative is added and it is stored in a cool, dark cupboard.

Gel support

The pH of the veronal buffer is adjusted to 6.6 with molar HCl. Agarose, 1 g, is dissolved by heat in 100 ml of this buffer. It is distributed in 10 ml amounts and may be stored at 4 °C for not more than 4 weeks.

Preparation of plates

Ten millilitres of agarose gel is melted and poured onto an 8×8 cm glass slide, using a levelling table if necessary. These plates will accommodate 27 tests. Holes are cut in the gel using a template (Fig. 1) and a cannula 3 mm in diameter, the plugs of agar are removed by suction.

Preparation of specimen

Most body fluids can be tested. Blood-stained or cloudy specimens are centrifuged and the supernatant is used.

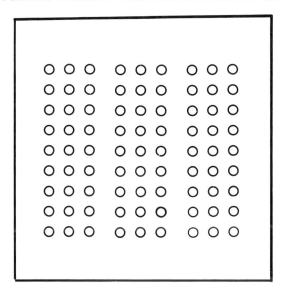

FIG. 1. Template for aligning the holes in the agar plate. (Actual size: 8 × 8 cm.)

Sputum: this is liquefied by adding an equal volume of 10% dithiothreitol and mixing on Vortex. It is then left at room temperature for 15 min.

Urines: these are centrifuged if cloudy or have visible debris, and then concentrated 20- to 50-fold using either ethanol precipitation or ultrafiltration. For ethanol precipitation boil the urine for 10 min, then spin at 3000 rpm for 5 min to remove coagulated protein. Five millilitres of supernatant is mixed with 15 ml of 95% ethanol and then centrifuged. The supernatant fluid is removed and the pellet is resuspended in 0.25 ml of distilled water (20-fold concentration). For ultrafiltration, the Minicon-15 (Amicon, Lexington, U.S.A.), may be used to concentrate urine 50-fold.

CSF: this is used untreated.

Lung tissue: this is cut into small pieces and ground in a Griffith or Ten Broeck homogeniser. The homogenate is suspended in saline, centrifuged and the supernatant fluid is used.

Antisera

Anti-capsular antisera (Statens Serum Institute, Denmark) are used to detect pneumococcal antigens. They are available as 'OMNI' serum reacting with 82 pneumococcal serotypes; group specific sera labelled A–I and monovalent sera. *Haemophilus influenzae* antisera are available from Wellcome or Difco laboratories as polyvalent and individual sera. Meningococcal and *Streptococcus* group B antisera are available from Wellcome as individual sera.

Electrophoresis

Antigen is placed in the cathodal well and antisera in the anodal well. A convenient volume for both reactants is 2 µl, delivered with a pipetting device using disposable tips. The agar plate is inverted onto the paper wicks to achieve a good agar-wick contact. A current of 200 V, 30 mA, is passed through the medium for 10 min. The plate is then removed and examined against an oblique light for lines of precipitation. If no lines are visible, the plate is reversed and returned to the tank, the current is reversed and re-applied for a further 10 min (Fig. 2).

Reading plates

Plates are examined for precipitation lines under a bright, oblique light. If the optimal of antigen-antibody has been reached, a sharp, straight line or arc will be seen midway between the two wells. Its location, thickness and shape will depend on the concentration of antigen in the sample and the potency of the antiserum. If weak or only faintly visible lines are seen with hand lens, the plates are placed in a moist chamber and left at 4 °C for 1 h, re-examined and, if still weak, they are left for a further 24 h at 4 °C. All apparently negative plates are treated in the same way.

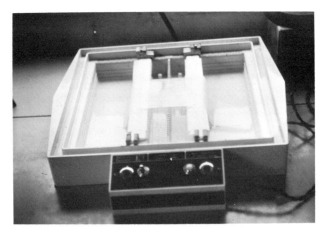

FIG. 2. Equipment for counter-current immunoelectrophoresis showing the tank, agar plate, wicks and buffer chambers.

Permanent preparations

These can be made with Gel bond (Miles Scientific). A thin sheet of clear plastic, hydrophobic on one side and hydrophilic on the other, is cut to fit an 8×8 cm glass slide. After electrophoresis, the agarose plate is immersed in phosphate buffered saline, the solution being changed several times. After 1 h, the plate is removed and the loosened agarose is floated onto another plate which has been covered with Gel bond with the hydrophilic side uppermost. The layered Gel bond is removed from the glass plate and placed between several layers of blotting paper, under a heavy weight for 30 min. By this time all moisture will have been absorbed, leaving a thin film on the plastic sheet which can now be stained with Coomassie Brilliant Blue R stain. For staining methods see the chapter by J. Longbottom and L. Taylor, p. 164.

Interpretation

CIE performance is affected by the quality of the agarose, the ionic strength of the buffer and the time of current application. The variations in thickness, shape and position of the precipitin lines depend on the source and specificity of the antisera, the lot to lot variation, the difference between polyvalent and monovalent sera and the amount of antigen present in the specimen. In high voltage electrophoresis, at optimal reaction, the precipitin line is visible after 10 min. Failure of reactivity can be due to lack of antigen, or lack of anodal migration due to the neutral or slightly positive charge of the antigen. This has been observed with pneumococcal antigens type 7 and 14. These polysaccharides can be detected with m-carboxyphenylboronic acid (Kelsey & Reed, 1979).

In some cases, immunoglobulins in the specimen or antiserum form a hazy or highly curved precipitate around the antigen or antibody well which may not disappear after dilution but may be eliminated by heating at 56 °C for 30 min to inactivate complement. Possible cross-reactions should also be taken into account.

Appendix: Applications

	Source
Antigen (*in vivo*)	
Bacterial	
Streptococcus pneumoniae	Sputum, serum, urine, CSF, pleural, joint, peritoneal fluids
All groups	
Neisseria meningitidis	CSF, serum, joint fluid
Haemophilus influenzae	CSF serum, urine, sputum, joint fluid
Pseudomonas aeruginosa	Serum
Klebsiella pneumoniae	Serum, CSF, urine, pleural fluid
E. coli K1	CSF, serum
Staphylococcus aureus (Techoic acid)	CSF, pericardial fluid
Streptococcus gp B	CSF, serum
Viral	
Hepatitis B surface antigen	Serum, tears, saliva, urine
Enteroviruses	CSF
Smallpox	Scab extracts
Protozoan	
Toxoplasma gondii	Serum
Pneumocystis carnii	Serum
Antibodies	
Bacterial	
Serratia marcescens	Serum
Staphylococcus aureus	Serum
Mycoplasma pneumoniae	Serum
Brucella melitensis	Serum
Fungal	
Candida sp.	Serum
Coccidiodes immitis	Serum
Histoplasma capsulatum	Serum
Actinomyces israeli	Serum
Aspergillus fumigatus	Serum
Viral	
Hepatitis B	Serum
Influenzae A_2	Serum
California encephalitis virus	Serum
Cytomegalovirus	Serum
Protozoan	
Trypanosoma cruzi	Serum
Amoeba histolytica	Serum
Trichinella spiralis	Serum
Leishmania tropica	Serum
Rickettsial	
Rickettsia quintana	Serum

References

BUSSARD, A. 1959 Description d'une technique combinant simultanement l'electrophorese et la precipitation immunologique dans une gel: l'electrosynerese. *Biochimica et Biophysica Acta* **34**, 258–263.

EL REFAIE M. & DULAKE, C. 1975 Countercurrent immunoelectrophoresis for the diagnosis of pneumococcal chest infection. *Journal of Clinical Pathology* **28**, 801–806.

GREENWOOD, D. M., WHITTLE, H. C. & DOMINIC-RAJKOVIC, O. 1971 Countercurrent immunoelectrophoresis in the diagnosis of meningococcal infections. *Lancet* ii, 519–521.

KELSEY, M. C. & REED, C. S. 1979 Countercurrent immunoelectrophoresis: Improved detection of pneumococcal capsular antigens in sputum by incorporation of a carboxylated derivative of phenyl boronic acid. *Journal of Clinical Pathology* **32**, 960–962.

MCINTYRE, M. 1978 Detection of capsulated Haemophilus influenzae in chest infections by countercurrent immunoelectrophoresis. *Journal of Clinical Pathology* **31**, 31–34.

PRINCE, A. M. & BURKE, K. 1970 Serum Hepatitis antigen (SH). Rapid detection by high voltage immunoelectrophoresis. *Science* **169**, 593.

The Application of a Novel Coloured Latex Test to the Detection of *Salmonella*

S. Gaye Hadfield, Nathalie F. Jouy and M. B. McIllmurray

Wellcome Research Laboratories, Langley Court, Beckenham, Kent BR3 3BS

Introduction

Latex agglutination tests have been applied to the detection of a wide variety of antigens and antibodies (Hechemy & Michaelson, 1984) and are popular in clinical bacteriology laboratories because they are inexpensive, simple to perform and give rapid results. The latex particles upon which the tests are based are uniform polystyrene spheres of microscopic size which can be coated or sensitized with antibodies (or antigens) by passive adsorption or chemical coupling techniques (Bangs, 1984). In conventional tests using white latex, the presence of the homologous antigen (or antibody) causes the sensitized latex particles to link together or agglutinate and the appearance changes from a uniform milky suspension to one of white clumps on a cleared background. Suspensions of particles of a colour other than white have been used but these offer no significant advantage. With these conventional tests, inexperienced personnel and sometimes experts, have difficulty in interpreting 'borderline' results.

Tests are generally used as probes for a single analyte. Multiple analytes may be sought if a suitable polyvalent sensitizer is used but cannot be differentiated without further testing.

The novel coloured latex tests described in this chapter involve the use of mixtures of latex particles of two or three different colours, where each colour has been sensitized with antibody of a different specificity (Hadfield *et al.*, 1987). In the presence of an antigen homologous with one of the antibodies, latex of a single colour agglutinates and the identity of that antigen is indicated by the colour of the agglutinated particles with a contrasting change in the colour of the background.

These coloured latex tests have several advantages over conventional latex tests:

1 Using one reagent, a single sample can be tested for the presence of up to three antigens, or mixtures of any two of the three; these are not only detected if present but are identified as well. This is particularly important when only a small sample is available.

Immunological Techniques
in Microbiology

2 The colour change which occurs when agglutination takes place is easy to read and interpret even in a borderline reaction.

3 The time taken for multiple testing can be considerably reduced.

The use of a three colour latex sytem has been explored in the rapid detection and identification of *Salmonella* to serogroup level.

Application of the Coloured Latex System to the Detection of *Salmonella*

Members of the genus *Salmonella* cause a wide spectrum of human diseases ranging from mild forms of gastroenteritis to severe, life-threatening enteric fever. Early, reliable identification of the organisms is important for the provision of appropriate therapy and the monitoring and control of outbreaks. The identification of salmonellae isolates currently demands a time-consuming battery of biochemical and immunological tests that in most clinical laboratories takes 3–4 days (see Fig. 1). Immunological tests, agglutination of whole bacteria with specific antisera, are used to identify the 'O', 'H' and Vi antigens of the salmonellae and, based on the Kauffmann–White scheme (Edwards & Ewing, 1972), the serotype of the strain can be determined. Very few clinical laboratories are able to identify all serotypes, as a large and unrealistic number of antisera would be required; most, however, are able to identify the common 'O' serogroup antigens and the Vi antigen. The 'O' antigens are typified by the repeating oligosaccharide units of the lipopolysaccharide components which extend out from the cell membrane to the surface. The Vi

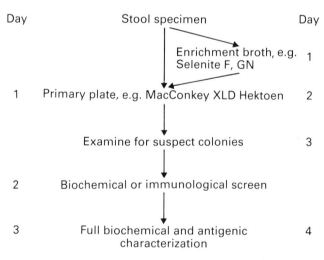

Fig. 1.   Typical isolation and identification of *Salmonella* from faeces.

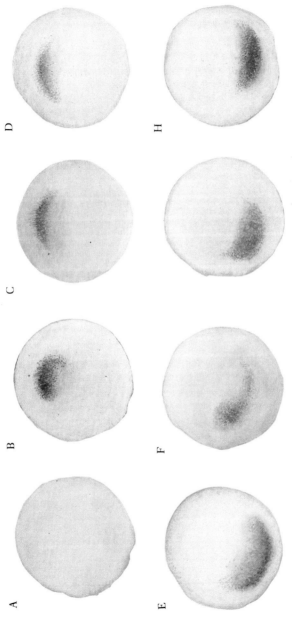

PLATE 1. Typical examples of the eight possible reactions obtained with *Salmonella* polyvalent latex. (A) Negative, (B) red, (C) blue, (D) green, (E) non-specific, (F) turquoise, (G) brown, and (H) purple agglutination. (i) Card mixed on a flat-bed rotator, and (ii) card mixed manually (*overleaf*).

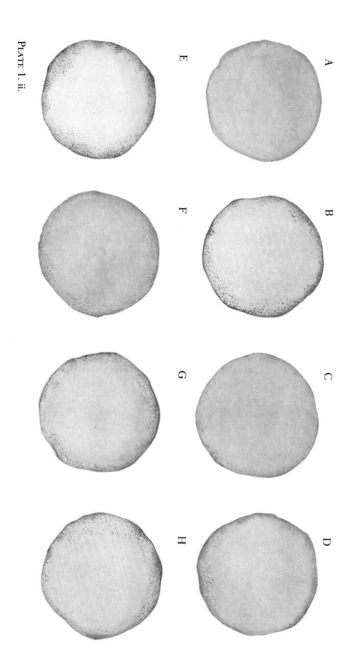

PLATE 1. ii.

antigen is a capsular polysaccharide thought to be associated with increased virulence, in particular with *S. typhi*.

The *Salmonella* coloured latex reagents, Polyvalent 1 and Polyvalent 2, have been designed to detect salmonellae rapidly and at the same time to identify the most common 'O' serogroups or Vi antigen. The composition of the reagents is shown in Table 1. Polyvalent 1 contains a mixture of red, blue and green latex particles which have been sensitized with immunoglobulins specific for 4–0, 6,7 and 8–0, and 9–0 respectively, representing serogroups B, C and D. In Polyvalent 2 Vi, 3 and 13–0, and 2–0 antibodies were used, covering serogroups A, E and G. Together the two Polyvalents will detect and serogroup approximately 99% of clinical isolates of salmonellae based on the incidence rates reported for the first half of 1985 in England and Wales. The eight possible results with each of Polyvalent 1 and Polyvalent 2 are outlined in Table 2, and examples of the reactions are shown in Plate 1.

In a typical test with an unknown strain, only one of the polyvalent reagents will react. For example, a suspension of *S. typhimurium* containing 4–0 antigens, would agglutinate the red particles in Polyvalent 1 which would separate from the rest of the mixture leaving a turquoise background; by contrast, none of the particles in Polyvalent 2 would agglutinate and the reagent would remain as a uniform brown/grey suspension.

The reagents are also capable of detecting and identifying mixtures containing two *Salmonella* antigens. For example the presence of both 4–0 and 9–0 antigens, as would occur with a mixed culture of *S. typhimurium* and *S. dublin*, would result in the agglutination of both the red and green particles of Polyvalent 1 which would appear as orange/brown clumps against a blue background. A mixed culture of *S. virchow* (6, 7–0) and *S. paratyphi* A (2–0) would result in blue clumps against an orange background with Polyvalent 1 and green clumps against a purple background with Polyvalent 2. Samples containing a mixture of *Salmonella* serotypes are relatively uncommon in clinical samples and consequently agglutination of two types of particle with a single culture will not often be seen.

There is an additional circumstance in which simultaneous agglutination of particles of two colours will occur; namely, with *S. typhi* strains which possess both 9–0 and Vi antigen. These are capable of agglutinating the green particles in Polyvalent 1 as well as the red particles in Polyvalent 2. With a fresh isolate, however, the Vi antigen usually masks the 9–0 antigen and Polyvalent 1 does not agglutinate unless the strain has been boiled to solubilize the Vi antigen and expose the 'O' antigen.

The Vi antigen is not exclusive to the genus *Salmonella*. To differentiate the other organisms from salmonellae and eliminate them from further investigation, when red agglutination is obtained with Polyvalent 2, it is necessary to boil a suspension for a few minutes, cool it to room temperature and retest with Polyvalent 1. Agglutination of the green latex will confirm *S. typhi* while other organisms such as *Citrobacter freundii* will not react and can be excluded.

TABLE 1.   *The composition of the Salmonella Polyvalent 1 and Polyvalent 2 latex reagents*

Colour of latex particles		Coating antibody specific for:	Latex detects serogroups	% of *Salmonella* isolated*
Polyvalent 1	Red	4–0	B	60.9
	Blue	6, 7, 8–0	C	17.3
	Green	9–0	D	15.6
Polyvalent 2	Red	Vi	*S. typhi*	2.0
	Blue	3–0, 13–0	E + G	2.8
	Green	2–0	A	0.7
			Total	99.3

* Figures reported for the first half of 1985 in England and Wales.

TABLE 2.   *Possible reactions obtained with Salmonella antigens and Polyvalent 1 and Polyvalent 2 latex reagents*

	Colour of agglutinated particles	Colour of background	Serogroup giving reaction with:	
			Polyvalent 1	Polyvalent 2
1	None	Brown/grey	Negative	Negative
2	Red	Turquoise	B	Vi
3	Blue	Orange	C	E or G
4	Green	Purple	D	A
5	Turquoise (green + blue)	Pink	C and D	A and E or G
6	Brown (green + red)	Blue	B and D	Vi and A
7	Purple (blue + red)	Green	B and C	Vi and E or G
8	Brown/grey (red + blue + green)	Colourless	Non-specific reaction	

Method of Use

The coloured *Salmonella* latexes have been used to:

1 Serogroup pure cultures of salmonellae.
2 Differentiate and identify salmonellae from other nonlactose fermenting colonies growing in mixed culture on primary isolation media.
3 Detect and identify salmonellae in primary enrichment broth cultures.

Colony identification

1 Pure colonies taken from nutrient agar plates or nonlactose fermenting colonies growing in mixed culture on selective plates (e.g. MacConkey, XLD, Hektoen, DCA) are removed by using the flat end of a wooden cocktail-stick. The number of colonies required depends upon their size: one or two will usually suffice but, as a rough guide, the quantity of growth required should be sufficient to cover the end of the stick (diameter = 2 mm).

2 The colony is emulsified in 200 μl of 0.85% saline using the cocktail-stick; an appropriate vessel for this is a well of a flat-bottomed microtitre tray. It is important that a uniform bacterial suspension is produced because clumps of bacteria can affect the appearance of agglutination patterns. The colony can not be emulsified directly in the reagent as this causes very rapid clumping of the homologous latex with entrapment of the other colours in the agglutinated matrix, giving the appearance of a non-specific reaction.

3 One drop (30–40 μl) of Polyvalent 1 is dispensed into one circle (diameter = 2.5 cm) on a white reaction card, and one drop of Polyvalent 2 is dispensed into another circle.

4 One drop (40 μl) of the bacterial suspension is transferred to each of the two circles using a Pastette (Alpha Laboratories, code No LW4282). It is important to dispense the latex before the bacterial suspension to ensure that the stock latex does not become contaminated inadvertently with bacteria.

5 A fresh wooden cocktail-stick is used to mix the contents of each circle, taking care to spread the mixture over the total area of the circle. A single stick can be used to mix the same suspension with both Polyvalent 1 and Polyvalent 2 reagents.

6 The card is either rocked by hand, using a gentle rotational motion, or placed on a flat-bed rotator, for 2 min. The rotator method produces clearer results and can increase the apparent sensitivity of the tests; the agglutinated particles appear as a concentrated spot in the centre of the circle surrounded by the appropriate contrasting colour. In order to achieve this pattern the rotator should have an orbital radius of 5/8″ (15.9 mm) and be set at a speed of 150 rpm (Wellcome Rotator, Wellcome Diagnostics, Dartford). To ensure that the agglutinated particles collect at the centre of the circle the surface of the card must be flat and the rotator must be on a level surface. If the card is not flat the particles collect at the edge of the circle, the same distribution as on cards rotated manually, compare Plate 1(i) and (ii).

Detection of Salmonella in broth cultures

1 Enrichment broths, for example Selenite F or Gram-negative broth (Difco), are seeded with a sample of a faecal specimen and incubated overnight at 37 °C. The

broths are formulated so that the salmonellae grow faster than other Gram-negative faecal bacteria.

2 The following day the broth is mixed by inverting the tube once after ensuring that the cap is firmly tightened. Steps 3–6 are followed as described for colony identification (above) replacing the bacterial suspension with the broth culture.

Conclusions

The novel coloured latex tests have been applied to the detection and partial identification of salmonellae. The tests are quick and easy to perform and the results are easy to read. Individuals with colour vision deficiencies cannot always identify the colour of the agglutinated particles but are aware that agglutination has occurred and can consult a colleague with normal colour vision. The two polyvalent latex reagents could replace both polyvalent and single factor 'O' sera as used in currently conventional procedures. The tests do not require pure cultures of salmonellae since they are not affected by the presence of large numbers of other enteric bacteria and therefore they have potential as screening reagents. The tests as at present constructed will only identify the isolate to serogroup level; if complete serotyping is required the results will enable more efficient use of conventional serological reagents. The principle of the coloured latex tests could be applied to the detection and identification of two or more antigens of any nature.

An additional embodiment of the principle is the combination of a single specific test latex with a control latex, where the control latex has been sensitized with immunoglobulin from an unimmunized animal. An example of this is a reagent to detect group A streptococci in throat swabs. This comprises a mixture of blue latex particles sensitized with immunoglobulin specific to group A streptococci and red particles sensitized with control immunoglobulin (Hadfield *et al.*, 1987). In the presence of group A streptococci the blue particles agglutinate, while non-specific reactions are identified by the appearance of purple clumps due to agglutination of both the red and the blue particles, against a cleared background. Non-specific agglutination of sensitized latex particles may have a variety of causes, including rheumatoid factor, strains of bacteria carrying protein A such as *Staphylococcus aureus* and extremes of salt concentration or pH. In conventional (white) latex tests a separate control latex is required in addition to the test latex to detect such non-specific agglutination.

In summary, latex-based tests provide rapid immunoassays. The novel use of mixtures of coloured particles increases the number of analytes which can be probed, makes results easier to read, reduces the time taken for testing, reduces the number of individual reagents and samples required and incorporates a built-in control with each test. The coloured latex tests could be applied to the detection of a wide range of analytes.

References

BANGS L. B. 1984 *Uniform Latex Particles.* Seragen Inc, PO Box 1210, Indianapolis, IN 46206.

EDWARDS, P. R. & EWING W. H. 1972 *Identification of Enterobacteriaceae*, 3rd Edn. Minneapolis: Burgess Publishing Co.

HADFIELD S. G., LANE A. & MCILLMURRAY M. B. 1987 A novel coloured latex test for the detection and identification of more than one antigen, *Journal of Immunological Methods* **97**, 153–158.

HECHEMY K. E. & MICHAELSON E. E. 1984 Latex Particle assays in laboratory medicine. Part 1. *Laboratory Management* June, 27.

The Use of Image Analysis to Study the Allergens in Foods

NEIL L. MORGAN, CAROL J. ALBERT AND KENNETH SPEARS
Department of Biotechnology, South Bank Polytechnic, Borough Road, London SE1 0AA

Introduction

General

Food allergy has received widespread publicity in recent years undoubtedly leading to confusion in the use of the term to describe other types of food intolerance. The term food intolerance embraces both allergic and non–allergic responses to foods and should be used when the underlying mechanism of the disease is unknown (see Fig. 1). For further details see Lessof (1985) and Pearson (1985).

Individuals suffering from food allergic disease show an adverse response to certain foods as characterized by an immunological reaction when the food is administered in a 'double-blind' challenge. This type of reaction is a form of 'destructive immunity' and is more common in infants and children of atopic parents. (Atopy is a hereditary disposition to allergic reactions e.g. eczema, hayfever, asthma) (Anon., 1984). The immunological reaction may be immediate or delayed and is frequently associated with a raised immunoglobulin E (IgE) level in the blood (Lessof *et al.*, 1980).

Diagnosis of food allergic disease

After an extensive patient history regarding reaction to foods has been documented, a number of different diagnostic tests can be used. The two most common are the skin test (Lessof *et al.*, 1980) and the radioallergosorbent test (RAST) (Wide *et al.*, 1967). The former involves pricking the skin and introducing the allergen usually in a 50% glycerol solution. The latter method involves coupling the allergen to a paper disc and detecting the presence of bound IgE by radioimmunoassay after flooding the disc with the patient's serum. The assumptions behind these tests are that all the potential allergens are present and that these are stable and active. Little attention has been paid to the careful preparation and evaluation of diagnostic solutions (Perlman & Ore, 1958; Morgan *et al.*, 1982). Failure to present all the

Immunological Techniques
in Microbiology

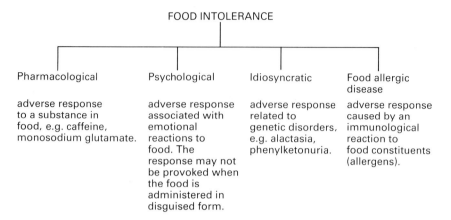

FIG. 1. Examples of food intolerance.

allergens in a challenge may result in false negatives. New techniques in protein analysis, such as crossed immunoelectrophoresis (CIE), enzyme-linked immunosorbent assay (ELISA) and protein purification, e.g. high performance liquid chromatography (HPLC), will assist in the preparation of good diagnostic solutions (Constable, *et al.*, 1982) which will ensure the accurate diagnosis of food allergic disease.

Special problems associated with food allergens

Reactions to food allergens may be immediate (e.g. observed in the mouth) or delayed and manifest themselves after absorption of the allergen. In addition, food allergens may be artefacts formed during food processing or formed as a result of digestion. All of these factors reduce the accuracy with which food allergic disease can be diagnosed. Other allergens e.g. grass and birch pollen and faeces of house dust mite do not necessarily pose the same problems.

There is some evidence to indicate that heating allergenic proteins reduces their allergenicity. It has, for example, been suggested that it may be feasible to produce a hypoallergenic infant feed from heat-denatured whey proteins (Kilshaw *et al.*, 1982; Heppell, 1984). Many food allergens are, however, glycoproteins which appear to be relatively stable to heat (Bleumink, 1970). The skin-sensitizing effect of allergens in legumes was shown to be reduced to varying degrees by heat processing (Perlman, 1966). New antigens have been shown to be produced as a result of pepsin hydrolysis of bovine milk proteins (Spies *et al.*, 1970), but this work has not been extended to allergens.

The allergenic proteins in cow's milk and eggs have been well documented but those in other foods are less well known; either due to their labile nature as in apple (Lahti *et al.*, 1980) or because they do not affect a large population.

Although it is possible for almost any food to cause an allergic reaction, it is those that are eaten more frequently which are most likely to produce these problems. Nuts were found to provoke an allergenic reaction in 22 out of 100 people (Lessof *et al.*, 1980), and it is likely that the level may increase with the increased popularity of vegetarian diets.

A wide range of nuts is eaten in the U.K. Peanuts (*Arachis hypogeaea*) are the most popular, although not a true nut but a legume. The other seeds that can be classified as nuts come from plants of different families, so it is likely that they contain different allergens. Brazil nut (*Bertholletia excelsa*) has been found to cause acute allergic reactions and is described as a potent allergen (Hide, 1983).

Sodium dodecyl sulphate-polyacrylamide gel electrophoresis (SDS-PAGE) has been used to study the proteins in peanut (Sachs *et al.*, 1981) but with the development of the new technique of immunoblotting it is intended to extend this approach to the actual identification of allergens. In this current work Brazil nut will be used as a model system but the techniques developed should find wider application in other foods.

Methodology

Extracts of brazil nut were prepared and analysed as shown in Figs. 2 and 3. Samples were taken during the process to check for intraprocess changes. Attention was paid to the starting raw materials in order to see whether batch-to-batch variation occurred, as this could affect the subsequent immunoblotting and interpretation of results.

Gel scanning

The image analysis system as used for gel analysis is still in development but it was realised that a potential existed for this system in microbiology/immunology laboratories. A number of interesting possibilities exist for this system. Namely:

1. Storage of gel scans on computer.
2. To analyse the gel images by enhancement and scanning.
3. To be able to produce a printed (hard copy) picture of a gel immediately so that no photography is needed.
4. To analyse published gel patterns and actually compare them to experimentally generated gels.
5. To write programs for the calculation of Rf values etc. automatically.
6. As the system measures levels of greyness in an image it could be applied to autoradiography.

The Sight Systems image analysing system is composed of a BBC 'B' or IBM PC microcomputer, a video interface system, a trackerball or mouse, a video camera

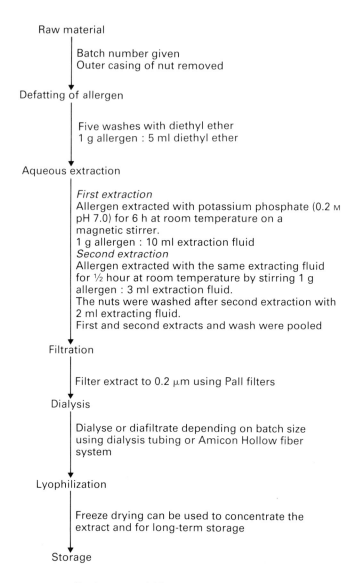

Raw material

    Batch number given
    Outer casing of nut removed

Defatting of allergen

    Five washes with diethyl ether
    1 g allergen : 5 ml diethyl ether

Aqueous extraction

    First extraction
    Allergen extracted with potassium phosphate (0.2 M
    pH 7.0) for 6 h at room temperature on a
    magnetic stirrer.
    1 g allergen : 10 ml extraction fluid
    Second extraction
    Allergen extracted with the same extracting fluid
    for ½ hour at room temperature by stirring 1 g
    allergen : 3 ml extraction fluid.
    The nuts were washed after second extraction with
    2 ml extracting fluid.
    First and second extracts and wash were pooled

Filtration

    Filter extract to 0.2 μm using Pall filters

Dialysis

    Dialyse or diafiltrate depending on batch size
    using dialysis tubing or Amicon Hollow fiber
    system

Lyophilization

    Freeze drying can be used to concentrate the
    extract and for long-term storage

Storage

Desiccator at 4 °C until use

Allergen extracts are stored and then analysed by SDS electrophoresis or isoelectric focusing and subsequently immunoblotted.

FIG. 2. Outline of allergen extract preparation.

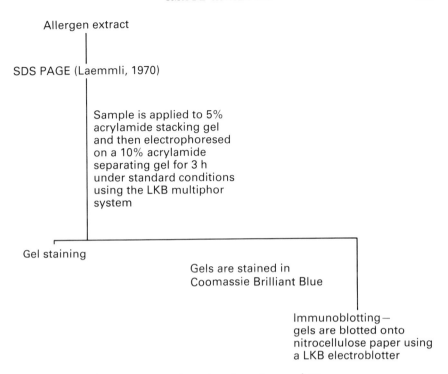

Allergen extract

SDS PAGE (Laemmli, 1970)

Sample is applied to 5%
acrylamide stacking gel
and then electrophoresed
on a 10% acrylamide
separating gel for 3 h
under standard conditions
using the LKB multiphor
system

Gel staining

Gels are stained in
Coomassie Brilliant Blue

Immunoblotting —
gels are blotted onto
nitrocellulose paper using
a LKB electroblotter

FIG. 3.   Analysis of allergen extracts: gel scanning using an image analyser.

(Hitachi CCCT Camera HV 720K), a high resolution monitor (Hitachi monitor VM 906E/K) and a large library of software (Fig. 4).

A large amount of memory is required for analysing video images. The pictures are not stored in the microcomputer but are held in the video interface system, resulting in virtually no use of the memory of the host computer.

Image analyser general description

The video interface peripheral (VIP) uses two video frame stores of 512 rows × 512 column resolution for image storage. Access to these images is via a high speed interface.

The system is driven by use of a mouse/trackerball and uses a menu area which occupies a quarter of the screen when required (Fig. 5). Each picture is stored as 512 rows and 512 columns of picture points, i.e. an array of 226 × 144 points.

The grey level resolution can be related to the number of bits in the store. A typical system would have six bits of grey store and one bit of binary store (64 levels). Seven bits of grey stores can be supplied as an option (128 levels).

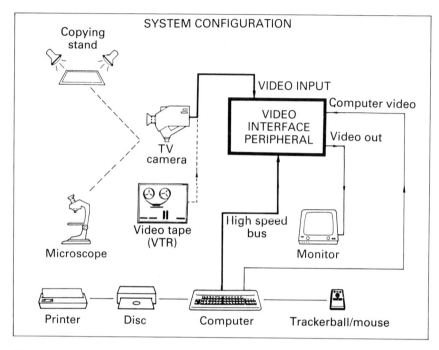

FIG. 4. Image analyser system: schematic.

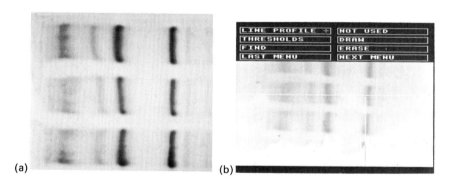

FIG. 5. SDS gel patterns of Brazil Nut extracts. (a) Photographed, and (b) image analyser profile.

The Grey and Binary framestores run at video rate, and have been designed to work in tandem. The Binary store is used for graphics and overlays which assist with measuring and picture processing.

After an image, e.g. a gel, has been correctly illuminated and a video picture has been frozen in the image analyser, the measuring procedure is followed.

The grey shade for each pixel is compared against the threshold setting and, if within limits, a white pixel is written into the binary frame store. This process is often called segmentation, detection or thresholding. It produces an image which is simpler to understand than its grey relative. The white binary image is overlaid on the grey image and is used to check precisely what will be measured. Video rate grey thresholding increases the speed of measurement and the ease of analysis of grey pictures.

The computer can read or write to any picture point (pixel) in the binary store, grey store or the menu area at any time. Computer picture access is continuous and no timing conflicts therefore arise. The computer controls every function within the VIP via a simple memory address structure. It is not necessary for the image to be frozen as the analyser can read a live image. The VIP is 'memory mapped' into the computer, thereby permitting simple, high speed software to be written.

Special software for gel scanning is being developed at the time of writing.

Other functions of the system are:

Object area measurement	Shape and feature analysis
X Y positions of objects	Movement tracking
Gel scanning	Autoradiography
Materials research	Multi phase analysis
Colony and cell counting	Dimensional measurement of objects
Direct printer dump of images	Computer storage of gel images.

In our laboratory, printer dumps of images have been used for colony counting on petri dishes. Other departments have used the system for movement tracking.

Gel scanning software

The custom software package developed for gel scanning operates in the following way: gel data is gathered from the picture along a horizontal line and stored on disc for use by the analysis program. Many lines can be scanned and averaged before storing. This technique helps to obtain truly representative data from the gel under analysis.

The analysis package uses a mixture of manual and automatic methods to find gel troughs.

Information on position, height and area for each peak is presented to the operator. The data can be printed or stored on disc as required. Using the manual method, the operator can decide upon the trough of the gel band. Using a screen driven cursor, a mark is left on the screen and the operator then finds the next trough. When all required troughs have been marked, data is available on the gel bands, i.e. the position, height and peak area. The automatic method requires good gel preparation to work totally automatically: with good gels no operator intervention is required.

Results

Figure 5a shows a typical photograph of Brazil Nut extract after SDS–PAGE electrophoresis. The same gel after scanning on the image analyser is shown in Fig. 5b. A single line has been drawn through the gel and a profile is shown at the bottom of the figure.

Further developments of image analysis systems will allow the recording and storage of gel patterns to be simplified.

Acknowledgments

We thank Dr M. Kemeny, Guys Hospital, and Mr S. Metcalf of Sight Systems Ltd, PO Box 37, Newbury, Berks, for useful discussions, and Sue Kingate for typing the manuscript.

References

ANON, 1984 *Food Intolerance and Food Aversion. A Joint Report of the Royal College of Physicians and the British Nutrition Foundation.* (Reprinted from the *Journal of the Royal College of Physicians of London,* April 1984, **18**).

BLEUMINK, E., 1970 Food allergy the chemical nature of the substances eliciting symptoms. *World Review of Nutrition and Dietetics* **12**, 505–570.

CONSTABLE, D. W., MORGAN, N. L., FOSKOR, A. P., ROOKE, M. D. & TAYLOR, W. A. 1982 *The Identification of Allergens in Conjuvac.* Abstract A314 International Conference on Allergy and Clinical Immunology, London 1984.

HEPPELL, L. M. 1984 Reduction in the antigenicity of whey proteins by heat treatment: a possible strategy for producing a hypoallergenic infant milk formula. *British Journal of Nutrition* **51**, 29–36.

HIDE, O. W. 1983 Clinical curio: allergy to Brazil nut. *British Medical Journal* **287**, 900.

KILSHAW, P. J., HEPPELL, L. M. J. & FORD, J. E. 1982 Effects of heat treatment of cow's milk and whey on the nutritional quality and antigenic properties. *Archives of Disease in Childhood* **57**, 842–847.

LAEMMLI, U. K. 1970 Cleavage of structural proteins during the assembly of the head of bacteriophage T4. *Nature* **227**, 680–685.

LAHTI, A., BJORKSTEN, F. & HANNUKSELA, M. 1980 Allergy to birch pollen and apple and cross-reactivity of the allergens studied with RAST. *Allergy* **35**, 297–300.

LESSOF, M. H. 1985 Food intolerance. *Proceedings of the Nutrition Society* **44**, 121–125.

LESSOF, M. H., BUISSERET, P. D., MERRETT, T. G., MERRETT, J. & WRAITH, D. G. 1980 Assessing the value of skin prick tests. *Clinical Allergy* **10**, 115–120.

MORGAN, N. L., CONSTABLE, D. W., FOSKOR, A. P. & ROOKE, M. B. 1982 *The Selection of Inhouse Allergen Extracts.* Abstract No. A317 at the International Conference on Allergy and Clinical Immunology, London 1984.

PEARSON, D. J. 1985 Food allergy, hypersensitivity and intolerance. *Journal of the Royal College of Physicians of London* **19**, 154–162.

PERLMAN, F. 1966 Food allergy and vegetable proteins. *Food Technology*, **November**, 58–65.

PERLMAN, F. & ORE, P. 1958 Allergenic extracts. A comparison of their quality and reliability. Description of technique for preparation of stabile allergens and proposal for biologic assay. *Journal of Allergy* **30**, 24–34.

SACHS, M. I., JONES, B. S. & YUNGINGER, J. W. 1981 Isolation and partical characterization of a major peanut allergen. *Journal of Allergy and Clinical Immunology* **67**, 27–34.

SPIES, J. R., STEVAN, M. A., STEIN, W. J. & COULSON, E. J. 1970 The chemistry of allergens. *Journal of Allergy* **45**, 208–219.

WIDE, L., BENNICH, H. & JOHANSSON, S. G. O. 1967 Diagnosis of allergy by an *in vitro* test for allergen antibodies. *Lancet* **ii**, 1105.

Quantitative Immunoelectrophoretic (QIE) and Immunoblotting Techniques Applied to Fungal Antigens/Allergens

JOAN L. LONGBOTTOM AND M. LOUISE TAYLOR*

Department of Allergy and Clinical Immunology, Cardiothoracic Institute, Brompton Hospital, Fulham Road London SW3 6HP

Introduction

The application of the various quantitative immunoelectrophoretic techniques to the identification and characterization of the antigenic mosaic of fungi and the interrelationships that exist between batches, strains, species and even genera has possibly been the most significant contribution in recent years to 'fungal immunology'. Complex antigenic mixtures can be quantitatively compared and characterized without the need for purified components, and fractionation and purification procedures can be monitored. By production of mono-specific antisera, the physicochemical characteristics of the specific component can also be determined. Furthermore, by using an allergic patient's serum and radiolabelled specific antisera (anti-human IgE) combined with autoradiography, specific components (allergens) can be identified within the complex antigenic mixtures. Similarly, components separated by sodium dodecyl sulphate—polyacrylamide gel electrophoresis (SDS-PAGE) or isoelectricfocusing (IEF) may be transferred electrophoretically or passively onto nitrocellulose membranes and, by applying appropriate sera/antisera, the molecular weight and pI (respectively) of particular components may be determined.

In this chapter, the quantitative immunoelectrophoretic (QIE) and immunoblotting methods as used in the authors' laboratory will be detailed and their application to the investigation of the antigens and allergens of *Aspergillus fumigatus* will be described. However, this is intended only as illustrating their potential use for all micro-organisms, whether fungal or bacterial.

*M. Louise Taylor was supported on a grant from the Medical Research Council.

Immunological Techniques
in Microbiology
0–632–01908–5

General Procedures

Preparation of antigen

For identification, particularly of allergens, it is recommended that the fungus should be grown on a chemically defined synthetic fully dialysable medium to avoid the possibility of contamination by high molecular weight medium-derived allergenic components. Thus, the choice of such a medium for optimal growth for each fungus (or bacterium) must be ascertained. For *Aspergillus fumigatus*, 'C. E. Smith's medium' (Smith *et al.*, 1948), an asparagine synthetic medium, originally used for growth of *Coccidioides immitis* and *Histoplasma capsulatum*, and similar to Sauton's medium for *Mycobacterium tuberculosis*, has proved to be satisfactory.

The fungus is inoculated into Thomson flasks containing 500 ml of medium (autoclaved 115 °C, 15 min) and allowed to grow in stationary culture, at 25 °C for 4–5 weeks. The culture filtrate is poured off from the mycelial mat (within a safety cabinet), sterile filtered (Seitz or membrane) dialysed (against running tap water for 24 h or four to five changes of distilled water, 10 vols to 1 vol of fungal extract at 4 °C for a 24–48 h period) and freeze dried. The mycelial mat is homogenized (Waring blender) in Coca's solution at 4 °C and then sonicated (MSE Soniprep) by repeated 5 min bursts at maximum power (with cooling in an ice bath to prevent overheating) until $\geqslant 80\%$ of hyphae are disrupted. The mycelial extract is then obtained by filtration, dialysis and freeze drying (as above).

Protein-enriched antigenic material may be prepared by saturation of the crude culture filtrate or mycelial extract (1 g/25 ml distilled water) with $(NH_4)_2SO_4$. The precipitate, allowed to form overnight at room temperature, is obtained by centrifugation and washed twice with saturated $(NH_4)_2SO_4$, redissolved in distilled water, dialyzed and freeze dried.

Depending largely on the titre of antibodies, 30–200 µg of antigen is optimal for most of the QIE tests listed.

Antisera

The most effective method for production of antisera in rabbits (N.Z. white or N.Z. white/Dutch lop cross bred) is by repeated subcutaneous and intramuscular injection of antigen. A 10–25 mg amount of extract in 2 ml saline is emulsified (by ultrasonication, MSE Soniprep) with an equal volume of Freund's Incomplete Adjuvant and injected (subcutaneously) into multiple sites. This is repeated after 4 weeks and thereafter the rabbits are boosted (intramuscularly) with a saline solution (2 mg/ml) until a satisfactory response, as determined on XIE tests (p. 164), is obtained.

High titre antisera from several rabbits (to overcome individual variations in antibody response) should be pooled for use as a reference antiserum. Sera should be stored at -20 °C. In XIE, for incorporation into the antiserum-containing gel, an amount varying between 7.5–15 μl/cm^2 gel is usually sufficient, although for weak antiserum up to 25 μl/cm^2 (and less antigen) may be required.

Monospecific antisera

The immunoprecipitin peak of the relevant antigenic component is excised from a number (8–10) of replicated, washed (isotonic saline overnight) XIE gels. These excised gel 'peaks' are then sonicated in a minimal volume of saline and emulsified with an equal volume of Freund's Incomplete Adjuvant. The immunization procedure for the rabbits is as above for the polyspecific antiserum, except that for the booster injections a saline 'gel sonicate' is used. The specificity of such antisera may be determined by the XIE-IG method (p. 167).

Human sera

Sera (obtained from clotted blood) from relevant allergic patients (i.e. skin test positive to the fungus under investigation) and control individuals should be stored at -20 °C.

Preparation of gels

The gel is prepared by dissolving agarose (Electran agarose 15; BDH, Poole, U.K.) 1 g in 100 ml diluted veronal (barbitone) buffer pH 8.6 (25 ml stock buffer $+75$ ml distilled water) by heating in a boiling water bath. The melted agarose is then poured onto a thoroughly cleaned (in chromic acid or boiling detergent) and precoated glass slide (8.2 cm^2) (coated with a thin film of 0.1% agarose and allowed to dry) or the hydrophilic side of Gel-Bond film, placed on a warmed level surface so that an even 1.2 mm layer of gel is formed (e.g. 7.5 ml buffered agarose per 8.2 cm^2 slide).

Electrophoretic conditions: for electrophoresis, the slide is placed in an appropriate electrophoresis bath, such that it forms a bridge between the anode and cathode reservoirs. The electrode compartments are filled with 1:2 dilution of stock veronal buffer, and wicks of filter paper (Whatman 3MM) or surgical lint are used to connect the slides into the buffer compartments. In this system, a suitable voltage for the first dimension electrophoresis for separation of antigen is 4 V/cm for 80–90 min and, under these conditions, no cooling system is necessary. It is advisable to check the potential drop across the gel plate with an appropriate volt meter. For the second dimension electrophoresis, at 90° to the first, and for fused rocket immuno-electrophoresis, a potential of 1–1.5 V/cm is applied (again checked) for 20 h or overnight.

Washing and drying of the gels: after electrophoresis the gel is washed overnight (24 h) in a bath of isotonic saline with 0.05% sodium azide, and finally dried with a layer of paper (Whatman 3MM), pressed evenly onto the gel surface (with rough side to the gel) and dried under a current of hot air from a hair dryer. When dry, the paper should lift easily from the surface.

For *crossed radioimmunoelectrophoresis* the plates are washed in three changes of the saline-azide solution, 30 min each, and dried by pressing three to four layers of filter paper (3MM) onto the slide under pressure (2–5 g/cm^2) for 10–15 min. The filter paper is then removed and the plates finally dried in a current of *cool* air.

Staining: the plates are stained in Coomassie Brilliant Blue R250 stain solution (0.5 g dye in 100 ml of ethanol: glacial acetic acid: distilled water, 45:10:45) for 10–15 min and then washed in successive changes of solvent mixture until the background is colourless. Care must be taken with the destaining so as not to decolourize weak precipitin peaks.

Quantitative Immunoelectrophoresis Techniques

Crossed or two-dimensional immunoelectrophoresis—XIE

For these tests, a single lower lateral well (3.5 µl capacity) is cut into the agarose for the antigen solution (10–60 mg/ml). After the separation of antigenic components in the first dimension, the slide is removed from the electrophoresis bath and a 'window', 3.5 × 5 cm, is cut out of the gel in the central area, the lower edge of this 'window' is approximately 3 mm from the antigen well and parallel to the first dimension migration (see Fig. 1A). A volume of 2.4 ml buffered agarose (as used to pour the gel) at 56 °C, to which an appropriate volume of antiserum is added and thoroughly mixed, is poured immediately into the 'window' and allowed to set. The slide, rotated through 90°, is then returned to the electrophoresis bath for the second dimension electrophoresis, ensuring that the direction of current is such that the antigen migration is into the serum-containing window area.

Although most protein antigens are negatively charged and migrate towards the anode at the pH used (i.e. pH 8.6), for detection of positively charged antigens a second antibody-containing gel 'window' may be placed approximately 3 mm below the antigen well and slightly closer to the cathode than the opposite gel 'window'. This 'window' technique avoids the somewhat tricky transfer of the first dimension gel from one slide to another, as recommended by others (Grubb, 1983; Ouchterlony & Nilsson, 1986) and ensures that not only is there good contact between the gels but also that the area of the immunoprecipitin peaks is free of any distortion, which can arise in carrying out the tests on smaller slides where they are not surrounded by an area of plain buffered agarose. This is especially important where changes in

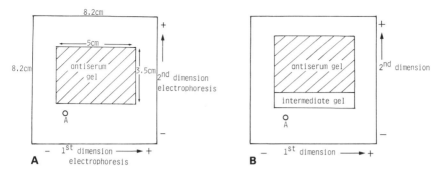

FIG. 1. A Scheme for XIE. Antigen is pipetted into the small well (A) for first dimension electrophoresis and then antiserum-containing agarose is poured into the 'window' made by removing an area of buffered gel (5 × 3.5 cm) for the second dimension electrophoresis. B Scheme for XLIE or XIE-IG. For the second dimension electrophoresis an intermediate gel (1 × 5 cm) incorporating either antigen or a second antiserum is placed between the antigen separation of the first dimension electrophoresis and the main antiserum containing gel.

antibody titre on serial samples of sera are to be determined (i.e. comparison of corresponding peak heights between two XIE tests) and also in XIE-IG and XLIE.

The concentration and volume of antigen, and the amount of antiserum used, is dependent on both the purity and strength of antigen and the titre of antibody. For *A. fumigatus* antigen, 3 μl of antigen at 30 mg/ml with 10 μl rabbit antiserum/cm^2 gel is usually optimal, (i.e. 250 μl antiserum + 2.4 ml buffered agarose for the 'window' gel), but for weaker sera less antigen and more antibody may be required to give adequate precipitin patterns within the 'window' area. Figures 2A and B are typical XIE tests of two different batches of *A. fumigatus* antigen (1 & 2) using a pooled rabbit antiserum.

Tandem crossed immunoelectrophoresis—TXIE

In this test two antigen samples in adjacent wells (5 mm apart, edge to edge) are run simultaneously in the first dimension. The resultant fusion of precipitin peaks is used to show the presence of common antigenic components within the two antigen samples. Also, since the height of an individual peak is proportional to the content of that particular component in the antigenic mixture, differences between the heights of the fused double peaks can be used to compare their relative amounts. Thus, different antigen preparations can be compared to a 'reference' preparation and batch-to-batch standardization achieved, at least for the major antigenic components, as in multicomponent systems identification of all fused peaks may be difficult. This is seen in Fig. 2C, i.e. TXIE of the two *A. fumigatus* antigens of Figs. 2A and B, where many fused double-immunoprecipitin peaks are present, some showing an increased height in antigen1 (indication of their higher concentration

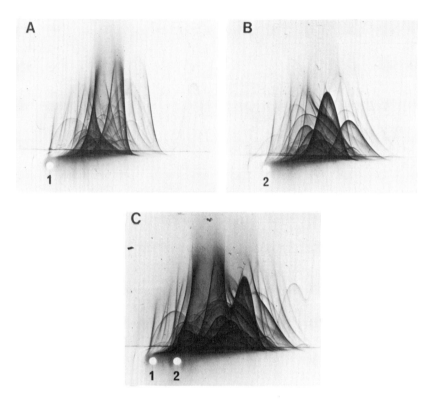

FIG. 2.   **A & B** XIE tests of two identically prepared culture filtrate extracts (1 and 2) of *A. fumigatus* against pooled rabbit antiserum. **C** TXIE of these two extracts.

in this antigen preparation) and others *vice versa*—a demonstration of the quantitative variation of antigenic components from batch to batch.

Crossed line immunoelectrophoresis—XLIE

For this test, an intermediate gel (1 × 5 cm) incorporating a second antigen (120 μg/ cm² gel) is placed between the separated antigenic components (of the first dimension) and the main antiserum gel window for the second dimension electrophoresis. This gel is poured as for (and before) the main antiserum gel by excising a gel window (1 × 5 cm) from the plate (see Fig. 1B) and pouring in the gel containing the antigen (i.e. 50 μl antigen, 12 mg/ml, to 500 μl agarose) allowing the gel to set, before removing the main window gel and proceeding as for XIE. Thus, by this technique, a direct comparison of the antigenic components within the two antigens may be made, since, in the antiserum gel, components common to the two antigens will form lines of 'identity' seen as a line-peak-line. Components unique to the electrophoresed antigen will remain as discrete peaks, whereas components present only in the intermediate gel antigen will appear as straight lines.

If excess antigen is incorporated in the intermediate gel, there will be complete absorption of its components as soluble antigen-antibody complexes and therefore only components (peaks) specific to the electrophoresed antigen will be revealed in the antiserum gel. This is known as XLIE with 'absorption *in situ*'.

XLIE is particularly useful in assessing qualitative differences between antigens—either in batches of antigen prepared for the same species/strain or in antigens prepared from different species within a genus or even different genera. This has been demonstrated for *A. fumigatus* where, in identically prepared culture filtrate antigens, although there appeared to be considerable batch-to-batch variation in biochemical properties and in immunological (antigenic and allergenic) activity, such differences were shown by crossed line immunoelectrophoresis to be quantitative rather than qualitative in nature (Longbotton & Austwick, 1986). Figure 3 shows that although the XIE profiles of two antigens appear very different (Fig. 3A and C) XLIE for each revealed no unique antigenic components (Fig. 3B and D). Further, the identity of a particular antigenic component in a fraction obtained by gel filtration was demonstrated (by XLIE) by the complete removal of a specific peak by 'absorption *in situ*' (Longbottom, 1986).

Crossed immunoelectrophoresis with intermediate gel—XIE-IG

An antiserum or serum to be compared with the reference antiserum in the main gel window is incorporated in an intermediate gel (1 × 5 cm) placed as in XLIE. For comparative analysis of the antibody content, a control test without antiserum in the intermediate gel must also be run simultaneously so that the heights of corresponding antigen/antibody peaks between the two plates can be compared. If antibodies are common between the two antisera, a reduction in their respective peak heights from those in the control plate will be observed due to 'absorption' by the antibody in the intermediate gel.

This method is ideal for testing the specificity of monospecific antiserum since only the relevant antigen peak should be 'absorbed' without any effect on the other immunoprecipitates. In Fig. 4 the specificity of a monospecific antiserum to a major *A. fumigatus* antigen (Harvey & Longbottom, 1986), produced as described above, is demonstrated by XIE-IG. The use of monospecific antiserum in the intermediate gel of fused rocket immunoelectrophoresis (FRIE) may also identify the component and give information on some physiochemical characteristics of the antigen, for example, its molecular weight.

Affino-crossed immunoelectrophoresis—AXIE

Incorporation in the intermediate gel of a suitable lectin either free or immobilized, e.g. Concanavalin A (50 μl 2 mg/ml in 500 μl agarose) or Concanavalin A (con A)

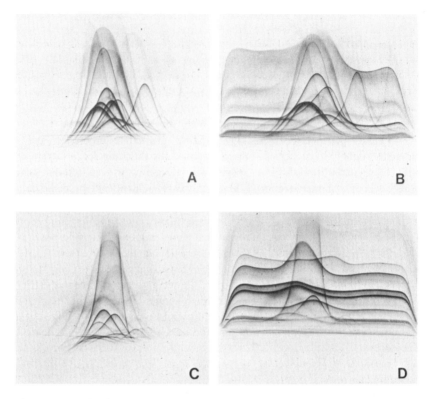

FIG. 3. XLIE tests of *A. fumigatus* culture filtrate extracts together with their individual XIE profiles. **B** XLIE of antigen in **A** with antigen as in **C** incorporated in the intermediate gel, and **D** vice versa. *Note:* no unique peaks remaining in either **B** or **D**, indicative of a quantitative rather than a qualitative (as might be expected from XIE profiles) difference in antigenic content between the preparations.

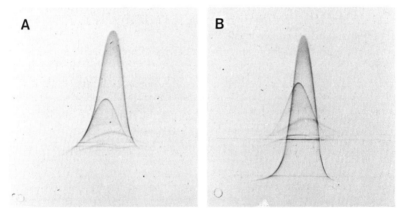

FIG. 4. XIE-IG to demonstrate the specificity of a monospecific antiserum. **A** control XIE of an *A. fumigatus* antigen fraction against rabbit antiserum and **B** with monospecific antiserum, raised to the predominant peak in **A** (produced as described in the text) incorporated in the intermediate gel. *Note:* absorption of only the one major peak without effect on the other antigenic peaks.

Sepharose may be used for analysis of terminal sugar residues of some glycoprotein antigens. By this method, many of the antigenic components of *A. fumigatus* were absorbed by the con A-containing intermediate gel, indicating the presence of terminal α-D-manno, or α-D-gluco pyrannoside residues and by employing autoradiography as for crossed radioimmunoelectrophoresis (XRIE, p. 170), their corresponding autoradiographs showed that most allergenic components were unaffected, indicating the absence of such end residues and suggesting a difference in the physicochemical nature of the major antigens and allergens (Longbottom, 1986).

Fused rocket immunoelectrophoresis—FRIE

This technique is particularly useful for the monitoring of fractions from column separation procedures as used for identification and purification of fungal antigens. Autoradiography, as described in the section on XRIE (p. 170), may also be applied for allergen identification.

In this test, buffered agarose (as for XIE) is poured onto prewarmed sheets (of appropriate size depending on number of fractions to be tested) of Gel-Bond (FMC Corporation) to form gels of 1.2 mm thickness. Areas of gel, e.g. 10×3.5 cm, are then removed and replaced to the same depth with buffered agarose (56 °C) containing antiserum. A series of antigen wells (1.5 mm diameter) are cut in a zig-zag fashion into the gel 5 mm below the antibody containing gel (according to a template placed under the Gel-Bond). These wells are filled with consecutive (or alternate) fractions obtained from separation, e.g. Sephacryl-S200 column or other systems, and allowed to diffuse for 1 h before applying the 'second dimension' electrophoresis (i.e. 1.5 V/cm overnight).

Figure 5 shows an example of FRIE applied to the Sephacryl-S200 column fractionation of the protein-enriched antigenic fraction of *A. fumigatus*. This showed that although most components were eluted as discrete peaks over relatively few fractions, some were eluted over a much larger number of fractions, indicative of a considerable heterogeneity in their molecular weights. The spread of antigenic activity was from $\geqslant 200$ kd to < 10 kd but the greatest number of antigenic components were eluted between 25 and 67 kd. On autoradiography (as for XRIE) there was a similar spread of allergenic components, with one major allergen, molecular weight 24 kd, being identified (Longbottom, 1986).

By incorporating monospecific antiserum to a specifically identified component into a 1 cm wide intermediate gel (10 μl/cm^2) placed between the antigen wells and main antiserum gel, the molecular weight of the component may be determined by reference to the elution curve obtained from molecular weight markers. Thus one major antigenic component, Ag 7, of *A. fumigatus* was shown to have a molecular weight of 150–200 kd (Harvey & Longbottom, 1986).

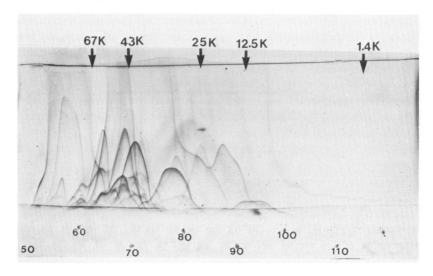

Fig. 5.   FRIE profile of a Sephacryl S200 column fractionation of *A. fumigatus* antigen.

Crossed radioimmunoelectrophoresis—XRIE

This method is used to identify those antigens within a complex mixture that are able to bind the specific IgE antibody from an allergic patient's serum—i.e. the 'allergens'.

XIE plates with antigen and homologous rabbit antiserum are run, washed and dried as previously described. A wax crayon border of approximately 1 cm is applied to each plate, leaving clear the central area with the immunoprecipitates. Then 3 ml of a 1 in 10 dilution (in phosphate buffered saline, PBS, pH 7.3) of an allergic patient's serum is carefully pipetted onto the central area of the plate (the wax crayon border confining it within the defined area) and left to react overnight (18–20 h) at room temperature. The plates must be on a level surface and also covered to prevent them drying up.

The non-bound serum proteins are recovered by gentle suction (with the plates slightly tilted) and the plates washed with 4–5 ml PBS at least five times for 10–15 min and blotted dry. Three millilitres of ^{125}I-anti-IgE Phadebas RAST isotope (Pharmacia Diagnostics, Sweden), diluted to approximately 100 000 cpm/ml in PBS containing 0.3% w/v human serum albumin (HSA) are then pipetted onto the slide and left overnight as previously. This method reduces considerably the volume of reagents, i.e. diluted serum and radioactive tracer, required as compared to other methods which involve placing the slide in a covered plastic box of the correct size and covering or immersing the whole XIE plate (Weeke *et al.*, 1983).

After carefully removing the non–bound anti–IgE (which may be stored at 4 °C for further experiments within 7 days), the plates are washed as before and finally dried in a current of warm air.

For autoradiography the dried agar surface of the plate is placed on X-ray film (DEF-2 Kodak Ltd) and left in the dark, under applied pressure for 5–7 days. The exposed X-ray film is developed by immersing in developer solution (Dental X-ray developer, (Kodak Ltd) diluted 1 in 4 in tap water) for 4 min at 20 °C, rinsed in tap water and then into fixer solution (Dental X-ray fixer, (Kodak Ltd) diluted 1 in 4) in two successive baths for 4 min each, thoroughly washed in running tap water and then hung up to dry. An increase in radiostaining intensity and faster development may be achieved by using X-OMAT L film (Kodak Ltd) and performing the autoradiography at − 20 °C together with a Du Pont Quanta III intensifying screen (Weeke et al., 1983). The XIE glass slide is stained as usual in Coomassie Blue. By comparing the autoradiograph with the XIE stained plate the allergenic components are identified as the antigenic peaks that bound the radioactivity and hence of specific IgE antibody. As well as individual tests with a number of sera from allergic patients to reveal variation of IgE binding components, tests should be included with sera from normal individuals and/or allergic patients not reactive to the allergen under investigation, in order to test for any non-specific absorption of either IgE and/or anti-IgE to the immunoprecipitates.

This method presupposes that in the immunization the rabbits have produced precipitating antibodies to all the allergenic components within the antigenic extract and that after immunoprecipitation in the gel, sufficient sites are still available on the potential allergen for reaction with the specific IgE of the patient's serum.

Studies of XRIE on A. fumigatus allergens using pooled allergic serum to demonstrate the broadest spectrum of IgE specificities have shown that, of the 32–42 precipitin peaks on XIE (depending on batch of antigen), 11–14 were identified as allergenic, 4–7 of which showed particularly strong radioactive uptake. A typical example of XRIE is shown in Fig. 6A and B, from which it can be seen that some of the strongest precipitin peaks are not allergenic i.e. do not bind specific IgE, whereas some of the peaks showing the most intense radioactive (and thus IgE) uptake correspond to peaks that are only poorly visible or even invisible with the protein stain (one such peak, which has been identified as a major allergen of A. fumigatus, is indicated).

The allergenic importance of the various antigenic components may be assessed by evaluating XRIE tests carried out with (10–20) individual allergic sera, in the form of an 'allergogram' which indicates the number of sera reacting (IgE) with each component. Thus components which bind specific IgE from at least 50% of the sera tested, with strong uptake by the majority, are defined as 'major' allergens, those to which less than 10% of sera show usually only weak binding are 'minor' allergens, while those falling between these two values are 'intermediate' allergens.

It has also been possible (Longbottom, 1983) to demonstrate binding of both

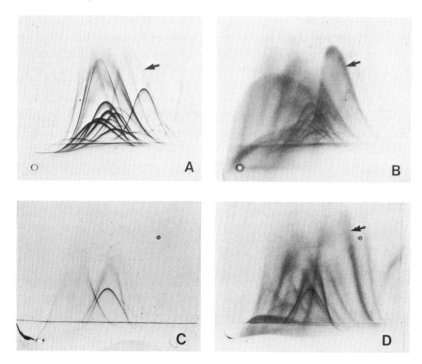

Fig. 6.   **A & B** XRIE of *A. fumigatus* using rabbit antiserum and a ABPA serum pool. **A** protein stained plate; **B** corresponding autoradiograph. **C & D** self-XRIE of *A. fumigatus* using the ABPA serum pool incorporated in the gel and as overlay. **C** protein stained plate; **D** corresponding autoradiograph. *Note:* not all protein stained antigen peaks show uptake of radioactivity, although for other antigens there is an increased sensitivity of the autoradiography as many peaks are not visualized by protein staining. This is especially noticeable in self-XRIE.

IgG and IgE antibodies, present in the serum of patients with allergic bronchopulmonary aspergillosis (ABPA), to some of the components of *A. fumigatus* by actually incorporating the patients' serum in the main window gel and proceeding as for XRIE—i.e. a self-XRIE test as shown in Fig. 6C and D.

Immunoblot-Analysis of Antigens and Allergens

This procedure involves the electrophoretic transfer of proteins/glycoproteins onto nitrocellulose membranes following electrophoretic separation by SDS-PAGE (sodium dodecyl sulphate—polyacrylamide gel electrophoresis).

Unlike XRIE, this method does not rely on rabbit antibodies to 'fix' the allergenic components, but depends on their migration in SDS-gel (hopefully without effecting the native antibody binding structure of the molecule although this may occur due to the mercaptoethanol reduction normally carried out, and even with SDS itself), and subsequent transfer onto the membrane.

Following transfer, the molecular weight of the components which are identified with class specific antibodies of either human or rabbit origin and visualized using specific enzyme or radiolabelled antibodies to human or rabbit IgG, is determined by comparison to molecular weight markers. Alternatively (although not detailed here) by passive transfer to the membrane of components after isoelectric focusing in agarose, the pI of components may be determined using the same identification methods.

Procedure

The antigenic extract is first separated on standard SDS-PAGE gels (Chapter 13), either gradient gels, or gels ranging between 10–20% polyacrylamide depending on the molecular weights of the particular components of interest—the higher percentage gels being required for lower molecular weight components, i.e. 20% gels for components in 10–25 kd range.

The antigenic components are then transferred onto nitrocellulose membrane (Trans-Blot Transfer medium, BioRad Laboratories). The gel, sponge pads (Scotch-Brite 6 mm), pre-cut filter papers and the nitrocellulose sheet (of appropriate size) are all equilibrated in 'blotting buffer' and then put (according to the manufacturer's instructions) into the Trans-Blot cell (LKB) containing transfer buffer (pre-cooled with tap water) and blotted overnight at 100 mA (approximately 10 V).

After transfer, unoccupied protein binding sites on the membrane are blocked by equilibration in 3% BSA (bovine serum albumin) in PBS for 2 h at 37 °C and washed three times in PBS with 0.5% Tween 20. The blotted SDS-PAGE gel and a reference gel with non-blotted samples are stained with Coomassie Brilliant Blue R250 (in methanol:acetic acid:water, 30:7:63) to evaluate the effectiveness of the transfer.

Immunological detection of particular components

The nitrocellulose membrane (possibly cut into strips for incubation with individual sera) is then incubated overnight with serum (poly– or monospecific rabbit antiserum or patient's serum, diluted 1 in 10 in PBS-Tween or PBS-Tween with 3% BSA) overnight at room temperature or at 25 °C for 2 h. After washing, five to six times in PBS-Tween, the bound antibodies are revealed with either isotope- or enzyme-labelled antisera.

Isotope labelled antibodies

For allergen identification after incubation in allergic patients' serum (i.e. IgE antibody detection) the membrane is incubated overnight in an appropriate volume of ^{125}I anti-IgE (100 000 cpm/ml, Phadebas RAST isotope, Pharmacia Ltd) diluted in PBS with 0.3% HSA, followed by washings (six times for 15 min each) in PBS-Tween.

For IgG antibody binding, (human or rabbit) ^{125}I-protein A (Amersham International) may be used in a similar way.

After washing, the nitrocellulose is cold air dried and placed against X-ray film (DEF Kodak) for autoradiography (procedure as for XRIE).

Figure 7 illustrates the identification of two strong IgE binding components, molecular weights approximately 36 kd and 18 kd, in a culture filtrate extract of *A. fumigatus*, using serum from a patient with allergic bronchopulmonary aspergillosis.

Enzyme-labelled antibodies

For IgG antibody detection, the membrane is incubated for 1 h at 25 °C with alkaline phosphatase conjugated anti-rabbit IgG or anti-human IgG (Sigma) diluted 1/1000 immediately before use in 3% BSA in PBS. After washing (as above) the membrane is incubated for 15 min at 25 °C with freshly prepared filtered mixtures

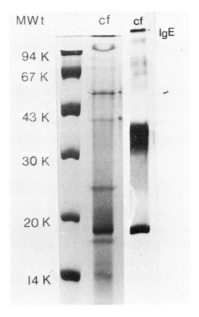

Fig. 7.   IgE immunoblot analysis of an *A. fumigatus* culture filtrate antigen, protein stained components together with molecular weight markers in left hand tracks, with the autoradiograph obtained using serum from a patient with allergic bronchopulmonary aspergillosis in the right hand track. *Note*: two major IgE binding components of approximately 36 kd (not strongly protein staining) and 18 kd.

of equal volumes of naphthol ASMX phosphate (Sigma) 0.4 mg/ml in distilled water, and fast red TR salt (Sigma) 6 mg/ml in 0.2 M Tris pH 8.2

For IgE antibody detection, enzyme-labelled antibodies, i.e. β-galactosidase anti-IgE (Phadezym RAST, Pharmacia) may be used, the chromogenic substrate being a mixture of 1.5 ml 2M β-D-galactopyranoside monohydrate (3.3 mg/ml in methanol), 1.0 ml Fast Blue B (20 mg/ml in PBS containing 20 µg MgCl$_2$.6H$_2$O/ml) and 7.5 ml of the same PBS. The membrane is immersed for 20 s and then placed on a filter paper pre-wetted with the substrate for 20–30 min at 25 °C.

Antigen/antibody binding may be semi-quantified using an appropriate scanner.

Appendix: Reagents

Asparagine synthetic medium (Smith *et al.*, 1948)

Seven grams of L-asparagine is dissolved in approximately 300 ml hot (50 °C) distilled water. Then, in turn, 7 g NH$_4$Cl, 1.31 g KH$_2$PO$_4$, 1.5 g MgSO$_4$.7H$_2$O, 0.9 g Na citrate and 0.3 g ferric citrate each dissolved in 25 ml distilled water are added to the hot asparagine solution mixing well after each addition. Finally, 10 g glucose and 25 ml glycerol are added and then distilled water to a final volume of 1 litre.

Veronal (barbitone) buffer (pH 8.6, 0.1 µM)

Stock solution contains 20.6 g sodium barbitone, 3.68 g barbitone and 0.1 g merthiolate in 1 litre of distilled water.

Coca's solution

Five grams of NaCl, 2.75 g NaHCO$_3$, 4 g phenol in 1 litre distilled water.

Phosphate buffered saline (PBS)

Eight grams of NaCl, 0.2 g KH$_2$PO$_4$, 1.135 g Na$_2$HPO$_4$, 0.2 g KCl, 0.2 g NaN$_3$ in 1 litre distilled water.

Blotting buffer

Seventy-two grams of glycine (192 mM), 15 g Tris (25 mM), 1 litre methanol (20%) and 4 litres of distilled water.

References

GRUBB, A. O. (1983) Crossed immunoelectrophoresis. In *Handbook of Immunoprecipitation-in-gel Techniques* ed. Axelsen N. H. pp. 113–124. Oxford: Blackwell Scientific Publications.

HARVEY C. & LONGBOTTOM J. L. 1986 Characterization of a major antigenic component of *Aspergillus fumigatus. Clinical and Experimental Immunology* 65, 206–214.

LONGBOTTOM, J. L. 1983 Antigens/allergens of *Aspergillus fumigatus.* Identification of antigenic components reacting with both IgG and IgE antibodies of patients with allergic bronchopulmonary aspergillosis. *Clinical and Experimental Immunology* 53, 354–362.

LONGBOTTOM, J. L. 1986 Antigens and allergens of *Aspergillus fumigatus.* II. Their further identification and partial characterization of a major allergen (Ag 3). *Journal of Allergy and Clinical Immunology* 78, 18–24.

LONGBOTTOM, J. L. & AUSTWICK, P. K. C. 1986 Antigens and allergens of *Aspergillus fumigatus.* I. Characterization by quantitative immunoelectrophoretic techniques. *Journal of Allergy and Clinical Immunology* 78, 9–17.

OUCHTERLONY, O. & NILSSON, L-A. 1986 Immunodiffusion and immunoelectrophoresis. In *Handbook of Experimental Immunology* 4th edn. Vol. 1: Application of Immunological Methods in Biomedical Sciences ed Weir D. M. pp. 1–50. Oxford: Blackwell Scientific Publications.

SMITH, C. E., WHITING, E. G., BAKER, E. E., ROSEBERGER, H. G., BEARD, R. R. & SAITO, M. T. 1948 The use of coccidioidin. *American Review of Tuberculosis* 57, 330–337.

WEEKE, B., SONDERGAARD, I., LIND, P., AUKUST, L. & LOWENSTEIN, H. 1983 Crossed radioimmunoelectrophonesis (CRIE) for identification of allergens and determination of antigenic specificities of patients' IgE. Chapter 32 in *Handbook of Immunoprecipitation-in-gel Techniques* ed. Axelsen N. H. pp. 265–272. Oxford: Blackwell Scientific Publications.

Aerobiology: Sampling and Detection Techniques

P. K. C. Austwick

Robens Institute of Industrial and Environmental Health and Safety, University of Surrey, Guildford, Surrey GU2 5HX

Jill A. Price* and Joan L. Longbottom

Department of Allergy and Clinical Immunology, Cardiothoracic Institute, Brompton Hospital, Fulham Road, London SW3 6HP

Introduction

Although antigens associated with airborne particles of respirable size are recognized as being responsible for a range of allergic disease, very little information exists on the airborne concentrations of these biologically active substances. An effect on health of such inhaled particles depends on their allergenic potential, the region in the respiratory tract in which they are deposited and the immune status of the individual exposed; for example, whether or not he or she is an atopic subject. The airborne particulate material involved varies widely in size, shape and origin; for example, as pollen grains, fungal spores or skin scales, but the underlying common feature is an antigen/allergen content which may provoke disease symptoms. It is also likely that the quantity of antigen/allergen inhaled correlates with the type and severity of symptoms, and a number of immunochemical assay methods, mainly radioimmunoassays, have now been developed for use on airborne particulate matter (Reed, 1982; Agarwal, *et al.*, 1983). This chapter describes two methods based on the ELISA technique for the assay of airborne material collected by five different sampling methods.

The choice of a sampling method depends largely on the amount of material required for the assay, the ease with which it can be removed or eluted from the collecting substrate, and the level of noise that can be tolerated during its collection. Particles may be collected by glass fibre or membrane filtration, impacted onto adhesive surfaces or washed (scrubbed) out of air by water spray, and the rate of air sampling can also vary from 2–2000 l/min depending on the instrument used.

Jill A. Price was supported on a grant from the Wellcome Trust.

Air Samplers

Air Sentinel (Fig. 1(a))

Technical data

Origin: Mayo Clinic, Rochester.
Size & Weight: 34 × 25 cm diameter, 8.2 kg.
Fan: incorporated, multistage *Airflow* 140 l/min.
Collecting medium: glass fibre filter 25 × 10 cm.
Particle cut off: 0.3 μm.

The Air Sentinel filters are dried to a constant weight before and after exposure and are therefore used for both total gravimetric determinations and estimates of airborne antigen/allergen. The advantage of this instrument is in its design for quiet running and the long, 72 h operation allowed.

Staplex Sampler (Fig. 1(b))

Technical data
Origin: Staplex Co, New York.
Size & weight: 28 × 23 × 37 cm, 5 kg.
Fan: incorporated single stage *Airflow* 1800 l/min.
Collecting medium: glass fibre filter 25 × 20 cm.
Particle cut off: 0.2 μm.

The Staplex High Volume Sampler is designed for use on industrial premises where noise levels are already high. It may be operated for up to 72 h and, because of its high airflow, it has been used for sampling in printing works etc., where a large sample of airborne material is required for the extraction of humidifier fever (HF) antigen.

Casella Personal Sampler (Fig. 1(c))

Technical data
Origin: Casella, London.
Size & weight: 12 × 7.5 cm, 0.58 kg.
Fan: incorporated *Airflow* 2 l/min.
Collecting medium: glass fibre 25 mm diameter.
Particle cut off: 0.5 μm.

The Casella Personal Sampler is worn on the clothing of the subject (the filter head may, for example, be attached to the collar with the battery in a pocket) and is designed to sample the air in the immediate environment of the wearer. It may therefore be used when the overall concentration of a component in room air does

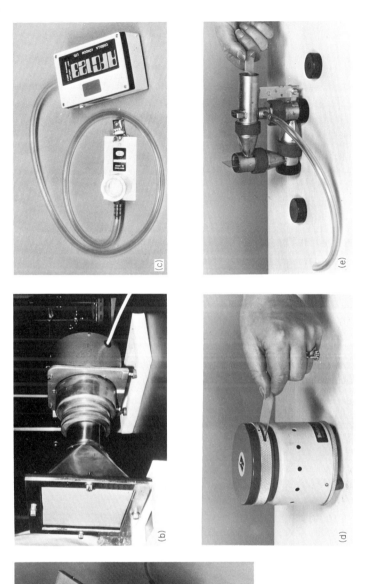

Fig. 1. Illustrations of the various samplers: (a) Air Sentinel, (b) Staplex, (c) Casella Personal, (d) Burkard Personal, and (e) Cascade Impactor.

not reflect the personal exposure of an individual and where contact with the particle source may vary in different areas. The rechargeable batteries run for 8 h on one charge.

Burkard Personal Sampler (Fig. 1(d))

Technical data
Origin: Burkard Manufacturing Co Rickmansworth.
Size & weight: 10×8 cm diameter, 0.5 kg.
Fan: incorporated *Airflow* 10 l/min.
Collecting medium: glycerol jelly.
Particle cut off: not known.

The Burkard Personal Sampler is a single aperture impactor, very quiet in operation and is compact and easily transportable. Particles impacted on the glycerol jelly may be examined microscopically or eluted for immunological assay. The rechargeable battery runs for 1.5 h at one charging.

Cascade Impactor (Fig. 1(e))

Technical data
Origin: Casella, London (No longer manufactured).
Size & Weight: 14×10 cm, 0.275 kg.
Pump required: capacity 40–60 l/min, e.g. Charles Austen F85.
Airflow: 27 l/min.
Collecting medium: glycerol jelly
Particle cut off: 0.5μm.

The Cascade Impactor was designed to fractionate the particulate matter in the air into four size-fractions. The largest particles are impacted behind the first aperture onto a glycerol jelly-coated full slide as a wide band of deposit. The three remaining sequential stages have similarly coated half-slides exposed to slit apertures of decreasing width but of standard length (17 mm), so that the speed of inertial impaction is increased to impact the smallest size particles caught at 0.5 μm diameter. The size range of the deposit is:

Stage 1   16–6.0 μm.
Stage 2   6.0–2.0 μm.
Stage 3   2.0–1.0 μm.
Stage 4   1.0–0.5 μm.

The running time depends on the concentration or the airborne matter or the drying-out time of the glycerol jelly. The slides may be mounted for microscopical examination or the deposit eluted for immunological assay. The chief advantage of the Cascade Impactor is that assay of the four size-fractions shows the distribution of allergen according to particle size.

Airborne Antigen/Allergen Quantification

The two methods described in this chapter are applicable to air samples in different environmental situations. The first, the sandwich ELISA, may be applied to measure levels of a recognized major antigenic or allergenic component, for example, the major Alt 1 allergen of *Alternaria alternata*. In particular, we have used it for major allergens associated with laboratory animal allergy. The second, the inhibition ELISA, is applicable to environments related to the group of diseases known as Extrinsic Allergic Alveolitis, where individuals have become sensitized to the environmental antigens and have mounted an IgG (usually precipitating) antibody response to inhaled antigenic material. Such diseases include humidifier fever (where as yet no causative micro-organism has been identified but an intense antibody response is seen to extracts of the microbial deposits known as 'baffle jelly', found within the humidifiers) or farmer's lung in which *Micropolyspora faeni* has been identified as the major causative micro-organism.

Materials and Methods

Antigen preparation

In order to perform either of the ELISA techniques described in this chapter for the determination of airborne antigen/allergen, it is necessary to prepare an extract containing the component(s) under investigation which will be present in an air sample. Dust collected from the area where sampling will be performed, or 'baffle jelly' in the case of humidifier fever, are good sources of this material and the specific components, once identified, can be separated from the extracted dust for use in the ELISA.

The dust (or 'baffle jelly') is extracted in Coca's solution (pH 7.2) for 48 h at room temperature, membrane filtered (0.45 μm pore size—Oxoid, London), dialysed against distilled water (48 h with several changes of water) and freeze-dried. The dried extract can then be stored in airtight containers.

Identified major antigenic/allergenic components (for example, major allergens identified by crossed radioimmunoelectrophoresis (XRIE) (see previous chapter) may be partially purified from the dust extract by Sephacryl S-200 gel filtration (Pharmacia, Uppsala, Sweden), and monitored by fused rocket immunoelectrophoresis (FRIE) (see previous chapter). Selected fractions containing the required antigen are pooled, dialysed (unless the fractionation has been carried out in 0.05 M NH_4HCO_3) and freeze-dried.

Antisera

Sandwich ELISA: for the capture antibody, antisera are produced in rabbits to the crude dust extract. For the detector antibody, monospecific antiserum is produced to the single specific antigenic or allergenic component which is to be detected/quantified (see previous chapter for methods).

Inhibition ELISA: human sera containing IgG directed against the environmental components are employed and should be of a titre sufficient to distinguish antigen concentrations to 50 µg/ml.

Purification of IgG

The IgG fractions of the rabbit antisera are prepared by caprylic acid precipitation (Steinbuch & Audran, 1969): 2.2 ml of caprylic acid (Sigma) are added dropwise to 25 ml of rabbit serum (diluted 1:2 with 0.06 M acetate buffer pH 4) and stirred vigorously for 30 min. The resulting solution is centrifuged (5000 rpm) and the supernatant removed and adjusted to pH 5.7 with sodium hydroxide. The precipitate, resuspended in 50 ml of 0.015 M acetate buffer pH 4.8, is centrifuged and the supernatant is added to the first supernatant. This is dialysed against 0.015 M acetate buffer at 4 °C overnight, then centrifuged and freeze-dried. The purity and activity of the IgG fraction is checked by immunoelectrophoresis against an anti-rabbit antiserum (Dakopatts, High Wycombe, U.K.).

Alkaline phosphatase conjugation of monospecific antiserum

For use in the sandwich ELISA, the monospecific antiserum directed against the component to be assayed, is conjugated with alkaline phosphatase (Voller *et al.*, 1976). Freeze-dried IgG fraction (1.4 mg) is mixed at room temperature with 5 mg (5000 units) of alkaline phosphatase (Sigma, Poole, U.K.) in 1 ml PBS and dialysed against phosphate buffered saline (PBS) at 4 °C for 18 h with two changes of buffer. Glutaraldehyde (8 µl) is added and incubated at room temperature for 2 h before redialysing at 4 °C overnight against PBS (two changes of 500 ml) followed by 24 h against Tris buffer (three changes of 500 ml, 0.05 M Tris/HCl pH 8.0). The resulting conjugates are stored at 4 °C.

Elution of antigen

The Staplex, Air Sentinel and the Casella Personal Sampler all collect particulate matter onto glass fibre filters which retain particles >0.5 µm. For antigen determination the complete personal filter (25 mm diameter), or for the larger filter

25 mm diameter punched out circles (for which a factor is incorporated into the calculation) are extracted by sonicating them in 1 ml PBS/Tween/gelatin buffer. If necessary, elution of the whole Air Sentinel or Staplex filter may be carried out by descending chromatography with NH_4HCO_3 (0.05 M), two or three eluates being collected, bulked and freeze-dried. After noting the total dry weight of the extract, it is reconstituted in PBS at concentrations ranging between 50–1000 μg/ml for use in the ELISA.

The Burkard Personal Sampler and the Cascade Impactor both sample onto microscope slides which are coated with glycerol gelatin (Sigma) and these samples are eluted directly from the slides with 1 ml PBS/Tween/gelatin buffer.

Measurement of antigenic activity

Sandwich ELISA (Fig. 2)

This is an adaptation of the double antibody sandwich ELISA (Voller *et al.*, 1976) and used for situations where the actual antigenic/allergenic component to be measured in the air sample/dust has been identified, and a monospecific antiserum to it produced. The IgG fraction of the rabbit antiserum to the relevant crude dust extract is dissolved in coating buffer (1 mg/ml) and 200 μl is added to each well of microtitre plates (NUNC Gibco, Uxbridge, U.K.). The plate is incubated at 37 °C for 2 h. After washing (200 μl PBS-Tween, three times) 200 μl of dilutions of the standard antigen and the extracted sample to be assayed (in PBS-Tween gelatin) are added and incubated for a further 2 h at 37 °C. (All tests are carried out in triplicate.) The plate is washed three times (as before) and 200 μl of the enzyme-labelled IgG fraction of the appropriate monospecific antiserum added and incubated at 4 °C overnight. This is followed by further washing and then addition of the substrate (200 μl). After 30 min at room temperature the reaction is stopped by the addition of 50 μl of 3 M sodium hydroxide and the absorbance is read at 405 nm using an automatic microtitre plate reader (Multiscan, Flow Laboratories, Irvine,

SANDWICH ELISA

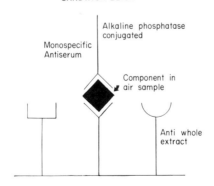

FIG. 2.   Schematic diagram of the sandwich ELISA.

CALCULATION

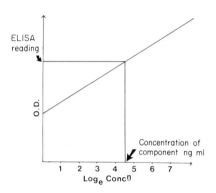

F IG. 3.   Typical standard curve for determination of antigen concentration by sandwich ELISA.

Scotland). The absorbance (optical density) obtained for the eluted air samples is read against the standard curve (Fig. 3) produced by plotting absorbance against $\log_e$ concentration of the standard antigen. The specific antigen in the air sample is then calculated according to the following equation.

Concentration of component in air sample (ng/m^3)
= Concentration of component (ng/ml)
× Total area of filter/Area of punched disc(s)
× 1/volume of air sampled (m^3)

Preferably several dilutions of the test antigen should be used and the mean value taken for the concentration of components in the sample. If the sample produces readings too high to read on the curve they will also need to be diluted, and this dilution must be taken into account when calculating the concentration of the component in the sample.

Inhibition ELISA (Fig. 4)

This assay may be used for situations where individuals have become sensitized to the environmental antigens and have produced IgG (usually precipitating) antibodies, for example in monitoring the airborne antigen in outbreaks of humidifier fever. Initially indirect ELISAs (Voller *et al.*, 1976) must be carried out in a 'chequerboard' fashion to determine the optimal concentration for the coating antigen and dilution of human serum. For an outbreak of humidifier fever, using a pool of sera from patients with strong precipitating antibodies to the humidifier 'baffle jelly' antigen extract, these were 25 µg/ml for the antigen and 1 : 1000 dilution of the human serum.

INHIBITION ELISA

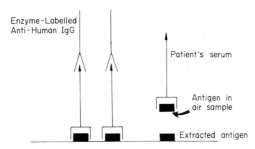

Enzyme-Labelled
Anti-Human IgG

Patient's serum

Antigen in
air sample

Extracted antigen

FIG. 4. Schematic diagram of the inhibition ELISA.

The microtitre plate (Dynatech, Billingshurst, U.K.) is coated with extracted whole antigen (25 µg/ml, 200 µl/well) in coating buffer at 4 °C overnight and then washed three times with PBS-Tween. For the standard curve, human serum (diluted 1:1000 in PBS-Tween) is incubated overnight with known concentrations (in the range 0–100 µg/ml) of the same antigen as that bound to the plate. For the test, the diluted serum is incubated with the eluted filter samples (50–1000 µg/ml). These samples are then added to the plate (200 µl/well) which is incubated at room temperature for 2 h. (To carry out the assay in triplicate, 100 µl amounts of standard or test samples are incubated with 600 µl amounts of diluted serum.) After washing, alkaline phosphatase-conjugated anti-human IgG* (Sigma) (1:500 PBS-Tween) is added and incubated for 2 h at room temperature. This is followed by washing, addition of substrate etc., as described for the sandwich ELISA. The concentration of antigen in the air filter eluate sample is read from a standard curve of absorbance vs $\log_{10}$ concentration of inhibiting extract. Optical density values for the air filter sample dilutions should lie on the linear part of the standard curve and the mean values for antigen concentrations are determined from two or three dilution values.

For measurement of levels of total allergen content rather than specific allergen in samples, a very similar method, although not detailed here, is that of RAST (radioallergosorbent test) inhibition. For this test the crude whole dust extract is covalently linked to a solid phase such as cyanogen bromide-activated paper discs or Sepharose particles (i.e. equivalent to coated microtitre plates) and human sera with high IgE levels to the relevant antigen is used together with ^{125}I-labelled anti-IgE. The assay is performed as above for the inhibition ELISA with the standard inhibition curve based on the percentage uptake of radioactivity rather than absorbance.

* As a radioactive assay ^{125}I-protein A can be used as a detector antibody (Reed, 1982).

Reagents

Coca's solution: 5 g NaCl, 2.75 g NaHCO$_3$, 4 g phenol in 1 litre distilled water.

Phosphate buffered saline (PBS) PH 7.4: 8 g NaCl, 0.2 g KH$_2$PO$_4$, 1.135 g Na$_2$HPO$_4$, 0.2 g KCl, 0.2 g NaN$_3$ in 1 litre distilled water. Adjust pH with glacial acetic acid.

Acetate buffers: 0.06 M (pH 4) 4.92 g CH$_3$COONa in 1 litre distilled water. 0.015 M (pH 4.8) 1.23 g in CH$_3$COONa in 1 litre distilled water.

Tris/HCl pH 8.0: 6.06 g Tris in 1 litre distilled water. The pH is adjusted with 6 M HCl added dropwise.

Coating buffer (pH 9.6): 1.59 g Na$_2$CO$_3$ (0.015 M), 2.93 g NaHCO$_3$ (0.035 M), 0.2 g NaN$_3$ (0.003 M) in 1 litre distilled water.

Washing buffer (PBS-Tween): 0.5 ml Tween 20 (Sigma) in 1 litre PBS.

Eluting buffers: (a) 1 g gelatin (BDH) in 1 litre washing buffer (PBS/Tween/gelatin), and (b) 3.95 g NH$_4$HCO$_3$ (0.05 M) in 1 litre distilled water.

Substrate: 1 mg/ml p-nitrophenol phosphate (Sigma Phosphatase Substrate) is added immediately prior to use to a stock solution of 9.7% diethanolamine (pH 9.6) in distilled water.

References

AGARWAL, M. R., SWANSON, M. C., REED, C. E. & YUNGINGER, J. W. 1983 Immunochemical quantitation of airborne short ragweed, *Alternaria*, antigen E and Alt 1 allergens: a two year prospective study. *Journal of Allergy and Clinical Immunology* 72, 40–45.

REED, G. E. 1982 Measurement of airborne antigens. *Journal of Allergy and Clinical Immunology* 70, 38–40.

STEINBUCH, M. & AUDRAN, R. 1969 The isolation of IgG from mammalian sera with the aid of caprylic acid. *Archives of Biochemistry and Biophysics* 134, 279–289.

VOLLER, A., BIDWELL, D. E. & BARTLETT, A. 1976 Enzyme immunoassays in diagnostic medicine. *Bulletin of the World Health Organization* 53, 55–65.

Immuno-Isolation Techniques for the Detection and Isolation of Plant Pathogenic Bacteria

D. E. Stead[1], J. F. Chauveau[2], J. D. Janse[3], M. A. Ruissen[4], J. Van Vaerenbergh[5] and J. W. L. Van Vuurde[6]

[1] *MAFF, Harpenden Laboratory, Harpenden, U.K.;* [2] *Service de la Protection des Végétaux, Angers, France;* [3] *Plant Protection Service, Wageningen, The Netherlands;* [4] *Department of Phytopathology, Agricultural University, Wageningen, The Netherlands;* [5] *Research Institute for Plant Pathology, Merelbeke, Belgium;* [6] *Research Institute for Plant Protection, Wageningen, The Netherlands*

Introduction

Most plant pathogenic bacteria survive from one crop season to the next as latent infections in propagating organs such as seeds, bulbs and tubers; in small pockets of diseased tissues such as cankers, or as epiphytic populations on plant surfaces. The populations of bacteria in these latent infections or on plant surfaces are often very low but they represent the primary source of inoculum for introduction of disease into subsequent crops. It is therefore necessary to have sensitive methods for their detection. The surfaces of plants normally contain a range of epiphytic and saprophytic bacteria, many of which are closely related to those species which cause plant disease. Any detection method must thus be selective. Most countries import and export seed and other propagating material. It is cost effective to maintain freedom from certain non-indigenous diseases and thus there are internationally accepted pre-export and post-import controls which include detection and diagnosis of latent and epiphytic organisms. Most methods rely on serology but isolation of the pathogen becomes necessary where confirmation is required.

Selective and semi-selective media are available for many plant pathogenic bacteria but most have poor recovery efficiency. Dilution plating on selective media usually provides the basis for detection but such methods are labour intensive and often impractical or too slow for effective screening of imported perishable material such as seed potatoes.

Immuno-isolation methods provide a potential alternative. The principles, methods and applications presented here form the basis of collaborative research and development projects to determine reliable methods for the detection and diagnosis of bacterial diseases of plants of quarantine or other statutory significance

Immunological Techniques
in Microbiology

within the European Community. They were the subject of two recent workshops; Wageningen in The Netherlands, and Merelbeke in Belgium.

Principles

Antibodies are absorbed onto a suitable solid phase and the remaining free surface is blocked with inert protein or with blocking agents such as Tween 20 or buffered glycine. This sensitized solid phase is placed in contact with the antigen (usually bacteria in comminuted plant tissues) so that the chance of collision of antigen with antibody is maximised. Plant debris and other bacteria are washed away. Non-specific and weakly bound bacteria are selectively desorbed and washed away. Finally, the strongly bound bacteria are desorbed and cultured.

A range of solid phases has been investigated and of these, polyvinyl chloride, polystyrene, nylon and cellulose nitrate provide useful substrates for antibody attachment.

Applications include:

1 Antibody-sensitized glass rods coated with cellulose nitrate (Van Vuurde & Van Henten, 1983; Van Vuurde *et al.*, 1986).
2 Antibody-sensitized plastic (PVC) Petri dishes or wells of microtitre plates (Van Vuurde, 1987).
3 Antibody-sensitized beads (agarose, nylon, polystyrene or cellulose nitrate coated glass) (Ruissen *et al.*, 1986; Van Vuurde *et al.*, 1986).

When populations of the target bacteria are low, desorption may be followed by (a) enrichment in broth or plant tissues before detection by plating, (b) symptom development in host plant, or (c) by another serodiagnostic method such as enzyme-linked immunosorbent assay or immunofluorescence (Hranitzky *et al.*, 1980; Van Vuurde *et al.*, 1986).

Immuno-isolation has potential uses other than the isolation of target bacteria from latent infections. Target bacteria may be isolated from media containing large numbers of other bacteria, for example infected tissues containing large populations of secondary invaders. Isolation of bacteria cross-reacting with antisera is useful for obtaining bacteria for use in monoclonal antibody screening tests or selective cross adsorption of polyclonal antisera. Immuno-isolation may also be used to quantify populations of target bacteria in quality control tests.

Methods

Basic procedure

This is based on that of Van Vuurde (1987).

1 Prepare the solid phase if necessary. Glass can be coated with a 33% (v/v) solution

of cellulose nitrate in acetone. Commercial nail varnish may be used. Glass rods may be prepared by heating the end in a Bunsen flame until partially molten and pressing it down on a flat surface to create an enlarged flat base. This stub is dipped into the cellulose nitrate preparation and allowed to air dry in an inverted position.

2 Coat the solid phase with antibodies diluted in a suitable coating buffer; for example carbonate buffer pH 9.6 as used for ELISA. Other coating buffers should be investigated and compared. It is useful to start with several different dilutions of antiserum. Coat for 1 h at room temperature or overnight at 4 °C.

3 Wash away unbound antibodies in a suitable buffer. Block unadsorbed surface with a non-specific protein. These steps can be combined by the use of 0.01 M phosphate buffered saline containing 0.1% Tween 20 and 2% bovine serum albumin (Clark & Adams, 1977), or quarter strength Ringer's solution containing 0.05% Tween 20 and 0.1% peptone (RTP). Carry out two 5 min washes.

4 Incubate with the test material. Incubation time and temperature will vary with the application. We normally incubate at room temperature for 30–60 min or overnight at 4 °C. The test material should be comminuted and suspended in the same buffer as the washings. RTP is recommended as it increases the rate of cell recovery.

5 Wash gently for 1 min in each of four changes of RTP.

6 Release non-specifically bound and weakly bound cross-reacting bacteria by washing for 3 min in each of two changes of low molarity (0.1–0.5 M) $CaCl_2$ or $MgCl_2$ in RTP.

7 Release strongly bound bacteria by a method suitable for the application, i.e.

(a) Rub glass rods over the surface of several plates of well dried agar media. Bacteria are physically removed from the rods.

(b) Break antibody-antigen binding by high molarity (1.0–2.0 M) $CaCl_2$ or $MgCl_2$ in RTP or low pH buffer and plate out.

(c) Break antibody-antigen binding by adding excess antibody or soluble antigen and plate out.

(d) Release by enzymatic breakdown of trapping antibodies with pepsin or papaine and plate out.

(e) Release by heat, for example molten agar in a poured plate.

Controls

Controls are required to test for non-specific binding of bacteria to the solid phase and to the protein layer. The following controls are thus considered essential:

1 Treatment of solid phase with coating buffer in the absence of antibodies.

2 Treatment of solid phase with pre-immune (normal) serum instead of antiserum.

3 Treatment of solid phase with antiserum against a non-homologous bacterium.

Extra controls should be included in the development of an application, although not all may be required for each test performed.

Development of test

The development of a method should begin with the use of pure cultures of the target bacterium. A comprehensive range of strains representing the taxon should be included. Recovery rates from a series of different bacterial populations should be determined. Samples of washings at each stage should be plated out to determine where losses may be occurring and, if good recovery can be obtained, the experiments should be repeated with mixed populations of bacteria. Finally, repeat with artificially infected material under a variety of conditions.

There are several potential limitations to any such method, the most important being antibody specificity. Antibodies which are particularly specific in one immuno-assay may not be useful in another and so it is wise to prepare antisera by a variety of methods and to test separate bleeds for each.

One solid phase may have a higher binding efficiency for one antibody molecule than for another and so it is recommended to test a variety of materials (Tijssen, 1985).

Once the antibodies have been adsorbed, the remaining surface should be blocked to reduce non-specific adsorbance. The choice of blocking agent may be important and a range of agents should be tested as for double antibody sandwich type ELISA. The optimum concentration of antibodies on the surface should also be determined. A range of coating buffers should be tested although the carbonate ELISA coating buffer, pH 9.6, is useful with polyvinyl chloride and polystyrene. The choice of washing buffer may influence the results and this should be taken into account. Any buffer used should maintain cell viability and it is necessary to test their effect on viability by plate counts. The incorporation of Tween 20 reduces non-specific binding. Washing may remove weakly bound target bacteria and plating out of washings will determine whether this is occurring. Any system using selective desorption must also take account of the loss of weakly bound target bacteria and the efficiency of the final desorption of strongly bound target bacteria. The various steps included may introduce other bacteria into the system and all reagents, including antisera, should be sterilized.

Finally, it is also necessary to consider a rapid method for identification of the target bacterium to determine plating efficiency in mixed populations. When molten agar is poured onto immuno-trapped bacteria, bacterial colonies may develop within the agar or between the agar and the solid phase even though they have been desorbed from the surface. Identification of such colonies is not always straightforward. Serological methods to facilitate identification of colonies on or in agar are being developed for several plant pathogenic bacteria (Van Vuurde, 1987).

Applications

Immuno-isolation methods including antibody coated rods, Petri dishes, microtitre plate wells and columns of agarose/sepharose beads are currently being developed and tested for the isolation of several plant pathogenic bacteria from naturally contaminated systems. These include:

1 *Clavibacter michiganense* subsp. *michiganense* causing bacterial canker of tomato.

2 *Clavibacter michiganense* subsp. *sepedonicum* causing ring rot of potato.

3 *Erwinia amylovora* causing fireblight of rosaceous hosts.

4 *Erwinia carotovora* subsp. *atrospetica* and *Erwinia chrysanthemi* both causing soft rot and black leg of potato.

5 *Pseudomonas cichorii* causing blight and leafspots in a range of different host plants including chicory, lettuce, chrysanthemum, tomato and pelargonium.

6 *Pseudomonas syringae* pv. *phaseolicola* and *Xanthomonas campestris* pv. *phaseoli* both causing important leaf spot diseases of beans.

7 *Xanthomonas campestris* pv. *pelargonii* causing leaf spot, wilt and stem rot of pelargonium.

References

CLARK, M. F. & ADAMS, A. N. 1977 Characteristics of the microplate method of enzyme-linked immunosorbent assay for the detection of plant viruses. *Journal of General Virology* 34, 475–483.

HRANITZKY, K. W., LARSON, A. D., RAGSDALE, D. W. & SIEBELING, P. J. 1980 Isolation of 01 serovars of *Vibrio cholerae* from water by serologically specific method. *Science* 210, 1025–1026.

RUISSEN, M. A., HELDERMAN, C. A. J., SCHIPPER, J. & VAN VUURDE, J. W. L. 1986 Selective isolation and concentration of phytopathogenic bacteria on immunoaffinity columns. In: *Proceedings of 6th International Conference on Plant Pathogenic Bacteria*, Beltsville, USA. The Hague: Nijhoff-Junk (In press).

TIJSSEN, P. 1985 *Practice and Theory of Enzyme Immunoassays*. Amsterdam: Elsevier.

VAN VUURDE, J. W. L. 1987 New approach in detecting phytopathogenic bacteria by combined immunoisolation and immunoidentification assays. *EPPO Bulletin* 17, 139–148.

VAN VUURDE, J. W. L., RUISSEN, M. A. & VRUGGINK, H. 1986 Principles and prospects of new serological techniques including immunosorbent immunofluorescence, immunoaffinity isolation and immunosorbent enrichment for sensitive detection of phytopathogen bacteria. In: *Proceedings of 6th International Conference on Plant Pathogenic Bacteria*, Beltsville, USA. The Hague: Nijhoff-Junk (In press).

VAN VUURDE, J. W. L. & VAN HENTEN, C. 1983 Immunosorbent immunofluorescence microscopy (ISIF) and immunosorbent dilution plating (ISDP): New methods for the detection of plant pathogenic bacteria. *Seed Science and Technology*, 11, 523–533.

Competitive ELISA, Co-Agglutination and Passive Haemagglutination for the Detection and Serotyping of Campylobacters

C. R. FRICKER AND R. W. A. PARK

Department of Microbiology, University of Reading, London Road, Reading RG1 5AQ

Introduction

Campylobacters are Gram negative, microaerophilic bacteria that are now recognized as a major cause of morbidity throughout the world. They have been implicated in a wide variety of clinical disease syndromes (Mandal *et al.*, 1984). It is the role of *C. jejuni* (and to a lesser extent *C. coli* and *C. laridis*) in the aetiology of enteritis and diarrhoea in human beings which has resulted in the intensive study of the genus during the last decade. During this time considerable progress has been made in understanding both the epidemiology (Blaser *et al.*, 1984) and the pathogenic mechanisms involved in the production of disease (Walker *et al.*, 1986). Much of our knowledge of the epidemiology of campylobacter infections is attributable to the development of schemes for distinguishing between strains. Aspects of the isolation and physiology of campylobacters have been reported in previous volumes of this Technical Series (Morris & Park, 1971; Skirrow *et al.*, 1982). Because of the inactivity of campylobacters in many standard physiological and biochemical tests, a wide range of typing schemes has been developed. These include schemes based upon resistance to various chemicals and dyes, possession of heat-stable and heat-labile antigens, susceptibility to bacteriophages, plasmid profiles, binding to lectins and analysis of restriction endonuclease patterns. All of these schemes have been of epidemiological value, but those based on the detection of antigens have proved most useful.

Several serotyping schemes have been proposed (Abbott *et al.*, 1980; Itoh *et al.*, 1982; Penner & Hennessy, 1980; Lauwers *et al.*, 1981; Lior *et al.*, 1982; Rogol *et al.*, 1982), but the two most commonly used are those described by Penner & Hennessy (1980) and by Lior *et al.* (1982). The Penner scheme uses heat-stable antigens of lipopolysaccharide detected by a passive haemagglutination (PHA)

Immunological Techniques
in Microbiology

procedure, whilst the scheme described by Lior is based on heat-labile antigenic factors detected by slide agglutination. When used in conjunction, these two serotyping schemes give a finer discrimination than either of the two systems used in isolation (Patton *et al.*, 1983).

When we became interested in the serological characterisation of *C. jejuni*, the Penner method of serotyping was already established in the U.K. This was due to the reference strains being readily available and, as there is no need to absorb antisera prior to use, the technique was relatively simple. Furthermore, the Penner serotyping procedure was published 2 years ahead of its main rival and had therefore been more adequately assessed. As both the Penner and Lior methods give adequate discrimination between strains, we have continued to use the Penner method on a routine basis. A further advantage of the system utilizing passive haemagglutination is that extracted antigens can be sent to reference laboratories for serotyping (Lastovica *et al.*, 1986) thereby overcoming the need to send live bacteria over long distances. This is particularly advantageous for campylobacters as they have a tendency to die rapidly. Furthermore, extracted antigens may be stored for periods of 6 months or more without losing their activity (Fricker, 1986). Thus, the procedure is suitable for reference laboratories and is particularly useful for epidemiological studies.

The Penner method of serotyping has much to commend it but it is labour-intensive and requires 24 h to obtain definitive results. We sought to improve the serotyping of campylobacters on the basis of heat-stable antigens by developing a method based on co-agglutination and by studying factors affecting the passive haemagglutination procedure. Another aspect of our work has been to use heat-stable antigens of campylobacters for detection of specific serotypes within cultures containing several serotypes so as to facilitate the search for specific types in epidemiological studies and so that results could be obtained rapidly.

Characteristics of the heat-stable antigens of campylobacters

The heat-stable (HS) antigens upon which the Penner & Hennessy method of serotyping is based were originally assumed to be lipopolysaccharide (LPS) in nature, because they behaved in much the same way as the 'O' antigens of the Enterobacteriaceae, in that they were extractable by EDTA or by heating in saline at 100 °C. Unequivocal evidence that the basis of serological heterogeneity was indeed lipopolysaccharide came from Mills *et al.* (1985). These workers used purified LPS to sensitize erythrocytes and showed that the results obtained with such antigen preparation were essentially the same as those obtained by using the original procedure of Penner & Hennessy. Furthermore, they presented evidence supporting the suggestion of Naess & Hofstad (1984a, b) that the LPS of *C. jejuni* is composed of lipid A, a core region and a short oligosaccharide side chain.

The Original PHA Technique For Serotyping
Campylobacter jejuni **and** *Campylobacter coli*

The technique was developed by Penner & Hennessy (1980). It involves four stages: preparing the stock antisera; obtaining heat-stable antigens from each test organism; attaching these antigens to red blood cells (RBC) and performing the haemagglutination (HA) test.

Preparation of antisera

New Zealand white rabbits are inoculated intravenously with live campylobacters of a reference strain, five times over a 2 week period. The bacterial suspension is prepared to an optical density of 0.375 at 625 nm and the volumes injected are 1, 2 and 4 ml; with further inoculations of 2 and 4 ml of a suspension containing double the concentration of bacterial cells. Blood is collected by cardiac puncture 7–10 days after the last injection. This is allowed to clot and the serum is stored at $-20\,°C$.

Preparation of antigens and sensitization of RBC

Each strain to be serotyped is grown on four blood agar plates for 24 h. The growth is harvested into 4 ml of saline and heated at 100 °C for 1 h. Following centrifugation, a 1:10 dilution of the supernatant fluid is used to sensitize an equal volume of a 1% v/v washed cell suspension of sheep RBC in phosphate buffered saline (PBS) (see Appendix). After 1 h at 37 °C the now sensitized RBC are washed three times and resuspended to 0.5% v/v in PBS.

Titration of antisera

Antisera are diluted in PBS to give initial dilutions of 1:40. Doubling dilutions (25 µl) of antisera are then prepared in microtitration plates with U shaped wells (Dynatech Laboratories Ltd). An equal volume of sensitized RBC is then added to each well, the plates are shaken, incubated at 37 °C for 1 h and stored at 4 °C overnight. Plates are then examined for haemagglutination. Absence of agglutination at the 1:40 dilution is taken as a negative result.

Modifications to the PHA Technique of Penner & Hennessy (1980)

One disadvantage of the PHA procedure as originally described is that it is labour intensive and usually requires 24 h to obtain a definitive result. The procedure can be shortened (Fricker *et al.*, 1987) to allow serotyping of campylobacters within 3 h.

Being nucleate, RBC of avian species sediment faster in haemagglutination assays than RBC of mammalian species. Both chicken and turkey RBC can be sensitized with campylobacter LPS antigens. Furthermore, chicken RBC sediment completely within 1 h whilst sheep cells (as used by Penner & Hennessy, 1980) require several hours for complete sedimentation. Thus the use of chicken cells in PHA assays considerably reduces the time required to obtain a result.

The time required for sensitization of erythrocytes with bacterial LPS antigens and the titre obtained is dependent on the antigen concentration (Neter *et al.*, 1952, Ley *et al.*, 1958). We investigated the possibility of reducing the time for extraction of antigens and subsequent sensitization of RBC. Using a bacterial suspension with an opacity equivalent to Brown's tube 10, only 15 min is required for each of these steps, thus reducing the time taken for serotyping by a further 1.5 h.

Whilst the combined use of chicken RBC and short periods of extraction and sensitization allows a considerable saving in time, there is further scope for improvement in the PHA technique. The number of serotypes recognized by the Penner serotyping scheme is now in excess of 60 and so, unless a screening technique such as the co-agglutination procedure described below is used prior to serotyping by PHA, a large number of titrations is required to determine the serotype of an isolate. The co-agglutination procedure is suitable for serotyping sporadic isolates, but when large numbers of campylobacters are to be serotyped, the technique has the disadvantage of requiring a different type of antigen preparation from the PHA technique, thus increasing the cost and effort of serotyping. We found that a slide PHA screening technique using a 5% v/v suspension of sensitized RBC gave almost complete agreement (315/316 strains) with the standard PHA technique. The aberrant strain was identified by the standard PHA procedure as serotype Pen 20/24 whilst the slide test was positive only with serum Pen 24. Only 17 antisera were used in this study and it is possible that other serotypes may not be amenable to study in the same way.

Protocol for Routine Serotyping of Campylobacters using Rapid Extraction of Antigens, Rapid Sensitization of Chicken RBC and Slide PHA

Preparation of antigens and sensitization of RBC

Growth from a blood agar plate is harvested into 0.85% saline, washed twice and resuspended to an opacity equivalent to Brown's tube 10. Antigens are prepared by heating the suspension at 100 °C for 15 min, centrifuging at 10 000 g for 5 min and collecting the supernatant fluid. A 1 : 10 dilution (in PBS) of the antigen preparation is added to an equal volume of 1% v/v chicken RBC (previously washed three times in PBS) and sensitization is carried out at 37 °C for 15 min.

The slide PHA procedure for screening of isolates

Sensitized RBC are washed three times in PBS to remove unbound antigen and are resuspended in PBS to give a 5% suspension. One loopful (about 3 µl) of the sensitized RBC is then mixed on a glass slide with an equal volume of each antiserum diluted 1:10 in PBS.

Haemagglutination is often immediately apparent but may take up to 1 min.

Confirmation of the result obtained by slide PHA

The 5% v/v suspension of sensitized RBC is diluted 1:10 in PBS and the cells reacted with the antiserum or antisera which gave positive results in the slide test. Twofold dilutions (1:40 to 1:5120) of antiserum are prepared in microtitration trays and an equal volume (25 µl) of sensitized RBC is added to each well. The plates are shaken and then incubated at 37 °C for 1 h by which time the RBC will have settled and the titre of the antisera for each strain can be determined.

Serotyping of campylobacters by co-agglutination

The principle of co-agglutination involves the attachment of antibody to particles which are then able to bind via the antibody to bacteria carrying specific antigens. Immunoglobulins in the IgG class bind specifically through their Fc portion to protein A, a substance present on the surface of some strains of *Staphylococcus aureus*, thus leaving the antibody-binding, $F(ab)_2$, part of the immunoglobulin free to react with antigen. Since many IgG molecules can bind to a single cell of *S. aureus*, agglutination of staphylococci and the antigen of interest can be detected when the two preparations are mixed together. The technique is generally more sensitive than direct slide agglutination, in which bacterial cells carrying antigen are mixed with serum, and is particularly useful when only a small number of specific antigenic determinants are present on a bacterial cell surface.

Since 1980 three groups of workers have applied the co-agglutination technique to the serotyping of *C. jejuni* (Kosunen *et al.*, 1980, 1982; Wong *et al.*, 1985; Fricker *et al.*, 1986). Kosunen *et al.* found that several cross-reactions ocurred with their co-agglutination procedure and that they could not obtain serospecific reactions with heat-stable antigens. Wong and colleagues on the other hand suggested that the type of co-agglutination obtained was indicative of the type of antigen involved in the reaction (i.e. whether the antigens involved were protein or LPS). Whilst we would agree that some reactions can be classified in this way, we have been unable to reproduce the results given by Wong *et al.* (1985).

Our co-agglutination procedure for serotyping *C. jejuni* and *C. coli* on the basis of heat-stable antigens (Fricker *et al.*, 1986) overcomes the problems of cross-reaction by using antisera raised against live bacteria, and bacteria heated at 75 °C for 30 min as antigens.

Preparation of antisera

The immunization protocol which we use is that described by Penner & Hennessy (1980) as outlined above. Rabbits are then test bled to ensure that they have produced antibody and are exsanguinated by cardiac puncture 7 days after the final injection. The blood is allowed to clot and the serum fraction is dispensed in 0.2 ml volumes and stored at -70 °C.

Preparation of reagent staphylococci

A Cowan I strain of *S. aureus* is inoculated into 1.2 litre of Tryptone Soya Broth (Oxoid CM129) and incubated at 37 °C for 24 h in a shaking incubator. Cells are harvested by centrifugation at 10 000 g for 10 min and washed twice with PBS. The cell pellet is then resuspended to 10% w/v in PBS containing formaldehyde (0.5%) and is stirred constantly at room temperature for 3 h. The cells are then washed three times in PBS, resuspended to 10% w/v and heated for 1 h at 80 °C. After a further two washings in PBS, the cells are resuspended to 10% w/v in PBS containing sodium azide 0.1% and stored at 4 °C.

Preparation of antibody-coated staphylococci

In order to save antisera and to limit the number of cross reactions it is necessary to use the antisera in a dilute form. To determine the optimal working dilution of antiserum, antibody-coated staphylococci should be prepared using various dilutions of antiserum. Doubling dilutions (1:2–1:16) of each antiserum are prepared in PBS. Undiluted serum (0.1 ml) and 0.1 ml of each dilution are added to separate 1.0 ml volumes of reagent staphylococci, mixed, incubated at room temperature for 10 min, and washed twice in PBS. The antibody-coated staphylococci are then resuspended to 10% w/v in PBS containing 0.1% w/v sodium azide and stored at 4 °C. The five preparations of antibody-coated staphylococci are then tested against their homologous antigen, prepared as described above. The staphylococcal preparation produced with the highest dilution of antibody which gives a strong agglutination within 1 min is chosen for routine use.

The co-agglutination procedure

A loopful of the antigen preparation is mixed with an equal volume of staphylococcal reagent on a glass slide and observed for 1 min for agglutination.

Value of co-agglutination for serotyping campylobacters

We found that over 95% of 400 campylobacter isolates gave serogroupings in agreement with those obtained by using the PHA technique. A small number of discordant results have been obtained.

A total of five strains gave a different serotype when tested by passive haemagglutination and co-agglutination, and a further 13 strains which we were able to serotype using passive haemagglutination did not serotype when tested by co-agglutination as described above. Of these 13 strains, however, seven gave concordant results when a more concentrated antibody preparation was used.

We conclude that the co-agglutination procedure which we have developed is a useful screening test for the serotyping of campylobacters although we always confirm the results obtained by passive haemagglutination. The method is particularly useful in situations where the number of isolates to be examined is low (less than 10 per week). The reagents are stable for up to 3 months at 4 °C which is a distinct advantage over the serum itself which must be kept frozen. Use of the co-agglutination system enables isolates to be serotyped rapidly so that infections due to the same serotype can be identified.

We suggest that the co-agglutination procedure is useful for serotyping of campylobacters, the serotype of which can be confirmed later by passive haemagglutination in batches of 40–50 isolates.

Competitive ELISA for the Detection of Specific Serotypes of C. jejuni

Due to the way in which some foods are processed, it is likely that several serotypes of campylobacters may be present in a given sample. Furthermore, campylobacters present in the environment may have originated from many sources and therefore be of several different types. It is thus necessary to have methods available for the detection of specific serotypes so that the possible sources of human infections can be identified. Serotyping schemes are important in such epidemiological investigations but their use is restricted to pure cultures and so only the most prevalent serotype in any given sample is likely to be identified. Lauwers *et al.* (1985) described a method for detecting multiple serotypes in poultry and human faeces. The method was based on 'selective killing' of certain serotypes with antibody and complement. Whilst the procedure appeared to be very effective, it is time consuming and may require several days to detect the serotype of interest.

We have developed a competitive ELISA system for detecting specific serotypes of campylobacters in foods. (Fricker & Park, 1986). The technique is relatively simple to perform and is applicable to organisms other than campylobacters. We shall therefore describe the procedure in some detail and give examples of its effectiveness.

Principles of indirect competitive enzyme immunoassays

This technique is based on the inhibition of the reaction of antibodies with immobilized antigen, by free antigen present in the test sample. The amount of antibody which binds to the immobilized antigen is inversely proportional to the amount of free antigen in the incubation mixture, i.e., the more antigen present in the test sample, the lower the amount of antibody which will bind to the solid phase, leading to a low enzyme activity. The antibody which binds to the solid phase can be quantified with enzyme-labelled anti-immunoglobulin antibodies.

As shown in Fig. 1, the presence of free antigen in the test sample reduces the amount of antibody which can bind to the solid phase. However this may not be the case if the amount of antibody added is greater than that required to completely saturate the antigen bound to the solid phase. It is clear, therefore, that the

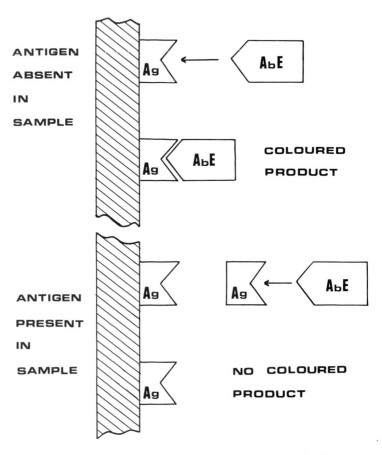

Fig. 1.   When antigen (Ag) is absent in the sample the Enzyme-conjugated antibody (AbE) binds to the antigen immobilized on the solid phase. Addition of substrate results in a coloured product. When antigen is present in the sample, the conjugate binds to this free antigen and is removed by washing so that the subsequent addition of substrate does not result in a coloured product.

concentrations of reactants need to be carefully controlled in order to obtain useful data. Furthermore, whilst proteins normally bind readily to polystyrene ELISA plates, polysaccharides bind less well. The problem has been overcome by developing methods to couple polysaccharides to proteins which adsorb strongly to ELISA plates.

The method we employ was first described by Gray (1979). Extracted campylobacter LPS is bound to poly-L-lysine via cyanuric chloride and the complex used to coat ELISA plates.

Preparation of antigen-coated ELISA plates

Campylobacters of a desired serotype are harvested from a blood agar plate into saline to a concentration 2.5 mg/ml total protein, determined by the Lowry method, using bovine serum albumin as a standard. The suspension is then heated at 100 °C for 1 h, centrifuged at 10 000 g for 5 min and the supernatant fluid is collected and held at 4 °C as stock antigen. Serial twofold dilutions (1:2–1:32) of the antigen solution are made in distilled water. Three glass test tubes are then prepared for each dilution of antigen, containing, (1) 1.0 ml of 0.01 M sodium hydroxide, (2) 1.0 mg cyanuric chloride crystals, and (3) 0.2 ml of 0.1% poly-L-lysine (molecular weight 30 000–70 000). The antigen solution is made alkaline by adding 0.2 ml of antigen to tube A. The contents of the tube are vortex mixed and added to tube B. Following a further vortex mix, the contents of tube B are added to tube C, which is then mixed and held at 4 °C for 2 h. The antigen-poly-L-lysine complex is then diluted to 10 ml with carbonate buffer (pH 9.6) and 100 μl is added to each well of a 96 well ELISA plate. The plate is then left at 4 °C overnight to allow adsorption of the antigen to the solid phase.

Determination of the antigen and antibody concentrations suitable for use in the competitive ELISA

The concentration of antigen bound to the solid phase has a marked effect on the sensitivity of the competitive ELISA system. As the concentration of bound antigen decreases, then the sensitivity of the assay increases. Nevertheless, as the results of the assay are read spectrophotometrically, it is necessary to have sufficient antigen and antibody present to give an absorbance in the range 0.8–1.2 for optimal sensitivity.

To determine suitable antigen and antibody concentrations for the assay, the antiserum to be used is titrated against each of the antigen preparations. Such titrations are carried out using antibody mixed with dilution buffer and antibody mixed with test antigen. The advantage of this is that the correct concentrations of bound antigen and added antibody for optimal sensitivity in the competitive assay can be determined simultaneously. The procedure is as follows. The antigen-coated

ELISA plates are washed three times with PBS-Tween (see Appendix). The remaining binding sites of the plate are 'blocked' by adding 200 μl of a 5% solution of horse serum in PBS to each well and incubating at 37 °C for 2 h. The plates are then washed three times with PBS-Tween. Dilution buffer (50 μl) is added to all wells of one plate, whilst test antigen (50 μl) is added to all wells in an identical plate. The test antigen is prepared by heating a suspension of 5×10^6 cells of the same organism used for preparation of the stock antigen, for 1 h at 100 °C. The suspension is centrifuged at 10 000 g for 5 min and the supernatant fluid is used as antigen. Serial twofold dilutions (50 μl in dilution buffer) of antiserum (1:1000–1:512 000) are prepared and titrated against each antigen concentration in the presence of either dilution buffer or test antigen. The ELISA plates are then incubated on a shaking platform (Flow Laboratories) at 37 °C for 1 h. After a further three washes with PBS-Tween, 50 μl of a 1:500 dilution (in dilution buffer) of alkaline phosphatase labelled goat anti-rabbit immunoglobulin (Sigma, U.K.) is added to each well and the plates are reincubated at 37 °C on a shaking platform for 1 h. The wells are then washed five times with PBS-Tween and 50 μl of a solution of para-nitrophenyl phosphate (Sigma) in substrate buffer (see Appendix) is added to each well. The plates are incubated at room temperature for 30 min and the enzyme reaction is terminated by the addition of 50 μl of 3 M sodium hydroxide to each well. The absorbance of each well is then read on a Microelisa minireader (Dynatech Laboratories Ltd). The corresponding wells on the plate to which test antigen has been added to those which give an absorbance of > 0.80 on the plate without added antigen are examined. Those wells which show a reduction of $> 50\%$ in absorbance represent conditions suitable for use in the competitive ELISA. Table 1 shows data from an experiment to determine the optimal concentration of reagents for use in detecting *C. jejuni* serotype Pen 1 by competitive ELISA.

The concentrations of antibody and bound antigen are selected and plates are coated with antigen at the appropriate dilution, placed in a sealed polythene bag and stored at -20 °C for up to 3 months.

Detection of campylobacters by competitive ELISA

Preparation of ELISA plates

ELISA plates are coated with antigen extracted from the desired serotype at an appropriate dilution as described above. Remaining antigen binding sites are then blocked by adding 5% horse serum (200 μl) to each well and incubating at 37 °C for 2 h.

Preparation of test antigen

Samples (10 g) are added to 50 ml of Preston enrichment broth (Bolton & Robertson, 1982) and shaken on an orbital shaker for 10 min. Solid material is

TABLE 1. *Determination of optimal concentrations of antigen and antibody for serotype Pen 1*

		Antibody dilution									
	Antigen dilution	1:1000	1:2000	1:4000	1:8000	1:16 000	1:32 000	1:64 000	1:128 000	1:256 000	1:512 000
Absorbance readings: no competition	1:2	118	118	116	113	110	108	106	93	81	56
	1:4	119	117	115	112	110	109	109	90	73	51
	1:8	113	111	107	103	100	98	94	89	71	50
	1:16	114	110	107	104	101	97	90	78	60	41
	1:32	110	104	100	91	81	70	63	51	39	33
Absorbance readings: competition with 'test' antigen	1:2	116	113	108	101	95	89	80	71	60	32
	1:4	115	110	104	96	89	83	74	61	50	26
	1:8	103	102	95	91	72	60	48	39*	29	21
	1:16	100	96	89	78	62	43*	37*	32	28	20
	1:32	92	80	63	51	31*	23	19	17	19	19

* The four readings marked with an asterisk satisfy the criteria of having an initial absorbance $\geqslant 80$ and giving a reduction in absorbance of $\geqslant 50\%$ when tested with competing antigen. The combination of an antigen dilution of 1:16 and an antibody dilution of 1:64 000 was chosen for routine use as this combination gives the greatest percentage reduction in absorbance when tested with competing antigen.

allowed to settle and the culture medium is removed and incubated microaerobically at 42 °C for 48 h. The enrichment culture is plated on Preston agar plates which are incubated microaerobically at 42 °C for 48 h. The remaining broth is centrifuged at 20 000 g for 10 min and the pellet is resuspended in 0.5 ml of saline. After heating at 100 °C for 1 h, the suspension is centrifuged at 10 000 g for 5 min and the supernatant fluid is used as test antigen.

The ELISA procedure

Antigen-coated, blocked ELISA plates are washed three times in PBS-Tween and 50 µl of each test antigen is added to two wells. Four wells containing 50 µl of saline are included on each plate. Two of these wells are used as negative controls (i.e. no antigen in sample) and the absorbance obtained with each sample is compared with the absorbance obtained in these wells to determine 50% reductions. The remaining two wells are treated with rabbit serum but receive no antirabbit immunoglobulin conjugate, and these are used to check that there is no non-specific binding of antibody to the solid phase.

Antibody (50 µl) at the pre-determined optimal concentration is added to each well and the ELISA plate is incubated on a shaking platform for 1 h. The remainder of the ELISA procedure is as described above, i.e. wash three times, add conjugate, incubate 1 h at 37 °C, wash five times, add substrate, incubate at room temperature for 30 min, stop the reaction by addition of 3 M sodium hydroxide and read the absorbance spectrophotometrically.

A well which receives no antibody or conjugate is used to 'zero' the spectrophotometer after addition of 50 µl of substrate solution and 3 M sodium hydroxide. The mean absorbance from the two wells used as negative controls (i.e. no test antigen) is obtained. Samples which give a mean reduction in absorbance of $\geqslant 50\%$ are taken as being positive for the particular serotype under investigation.

To date we have used the ELISA system to look for four different serotypes in 200 food samples. The results obtained are given in Table 2 which shows that the ELISA procedure is more effective at detecting specific serotypes than the serotyping of four colonies obtained on solid media. The system, however, is designed for detecting a specific serotype in naturally contaminated materials, for example during source tracing in epidemiological investigations. It is not practical to attempt to use the competitive ELISA system for detecting all campylobacters in any given sample.

The competitive ELISA system is a relatively straightforward procedure which can be applied to many situations. Whilst we have used it during our work with campylobacters, the system as we have described it could be used with any Gram negative organism. A similar system has been used to good effect for the detection of LPS antigens of salmonellas in poultry samples (Rigby, 1984).

TABLE 2. *Detection of serotypes Pen, 2, 3 and 4 in 200 meat samples by culture and competitive ELISA**

| | Positive for | | | |
	Pen 1	Pen 2	Pen 3	Pen 4
Culture	68	92	31	29
ELISA	91	128	43	37

* No sample was positive for any of the four serotypes by culture and negative by ELISA.

The Promise of Monoclonal Antibodies

Whilst our work with monoclonal antibodies is not described in this chapter, we have found that such antibodies are extremely useful in overcoming some of the problems which we have faced. Using mice immunized with purified campylobacter LPS we have prepared hybridomas producing antibodies which are specific for serotypes Pen 1, Pen 2 and Pen 3. We have used these antibodies in our co-agglutination procedure and the preliminary results are encouraging. Furthermore the use of these same antibodies has allowed us to develop a sandwich ELISA system for detecting Pen 1, Pen 2 and Pen 3 in naturally contaminated materials. The production of monoclonal antibodies is a relatively simple procedure and many laboratories have facilities for this type of work. We are convinced that the application of monoclonal antibody technology to the problem of serotyping campylobacters will result in simpler and more unified procedures being developed for use worldwide.

Acknowledgements

We would like to thank Mrs Sue Tompsett for technical assistance. The financial support of the Ministry of Agriculture, Fisheries and Food is gratefully acknowledged.

Appendix

Media

Preston enrichment broth

Nutrient broth No. 2 (Oxoid CM67)	500 ml
Saponin lysed horse blood	25 ml
Antibiotic solution	5 ml
FBP supplement	2 ml

Preston agar

As for Preston enrichment broth but with 1.2% New Zealand agar.

FBP supplement

Sodium pyruvate	12.5 g
Sodium metabisulphite	12.5 g
Ferrous sulphate heptahydrate	12.5 g

Dissolve in distilled water to 100 ml, sterilize by membrane filtration and dispense in 2 ml volumes. Store at -20 °C.

Antibiotic solution for Preston media

Rifampicin 100 mg dissolved in 25 ml methanol.
Trimethoprim 100 mg and polymyxin B sulphate 50 000 international units dissolved in 60 ml of distilled water.
Mix the two solutions, make up to 100 ml and sterilize by membrane filtration. Dispense in 5 ml volumes and store at -20 °C.

ELISA reagents

Carbonate coating buffer

0.05 M sodium carbonate pH 9.6 containing 0.02% sodium azide.

Phosphate buffered saline

Sodium chloride 8.0 g, potassium chloride 0.2 g, potassium dihydrogen phosphate 0.2 g and disodium hydrogen phosphate 1.15 g. Make up to 1 litre with distilled water.

Blocking buffer

Sterile horse serum (5%) in PBS containing 0.5% Tween 20.

Dilution buffer

PBS containing 0.05% Tween 20.

Substrate solution

P-nitrophenyl phosphate (Sigma) — 1 mg in 9.7% v/v diethylamine containing 0.02% sodium azide and adjusted to pH 9.8 with hydrochloric acid. The buffer can be prepared in bulk and stored at 4 °C. Tablets containing 5 mg of p-nitrophenyl phosphate can be purchased from Sigma and must be stored at -20 °C.

References

ABBOTT, J. D., DALE, B. A. S., ELDRIDGE, J., JONES, D. M. & SUTCLIFFE, E. 1980 Serotyping of *Campylobacter jejuni/coli. Journal of Clinical Pathology* 33, 762–766.

BLASER, M. J., TAYLOR, D. N. & FELDMAN, R. A. 1984 Epidemiology of *Campylobacter* infections. In *Campylobacter Infection in Man and Animals* ed. Butzler, J. P. pp. 143–161. Florida: CRC Press.

BOLTON, F. J. & ROBERTSON, L. 1982 A selective medium for isolating *Campylobacter jejuni/coli. Journal of Clinical Pathology* 35, 462–467.

FRICKER, C. R. 1986 Campylobacter serotyping on shipped antigen extracts. *Lancet* i, 554.

FRICKER, C. R., ALEMOHAMMAD, M. M. & PARK R. W. A. 1987 A study of factors affecting the sensitivity of the passive haemagglutination method for serotyping *Campylobacter jejuni* and *Campylobacter coli*, and recommendations for a more rapid procedure. *Canadian Journal of Microbiology* 33, 33–39.

FRICKER, C. R. & PARK, R. W. A. 1986 Enzyme-linked immunoassay for detection of campylobacters in foods. In *Proceedings of the Second World Congress on Foodborne Infections and Intoxications* pp. 111–113.

FRICKER, C. R., URADZINSKI, J., ALEMOHAMMAD, M. M., PARK, R. W. A., WHELAN, C. & GIRDWOOD, R. W. A. 1986 Serotyping of campylobacters by co-agglutination on the basis of heat-stable antigens. *Journal of Medical Microbiology* 21, 83–86.

GRAY, B. M. 1979 ELISA methodology for polysaccharide antigens: protein coupling of polysaccharide for adsorption to plastic tubes. *Journal of Immunological Methods* 28, 187–192.

ITOH, T., SAITO, K., YANAGAWA, Y., SAKAI, S. & OHASHI, M. 1982 Serological typing of thermophilic campylobacters isolated in Tokyo. In *Campylobacter: Epidemiology, Pathogenesis and Biochemistry* ed. Newell, D. G. pp. 106–110. Lancaster: MTP Press.

KOSUNEN, T. U., DANIELSSON, D. & KJELLANDER, J. 1980 Serology of *Campylobacter fetus ss. jejuni* (related campylobacters). Demonstration of strain specific and interstrain-related antigens by immunoelectrophoresis and co-agglutination. *Acta Pathologica, Microbiologica et Immunologica Scandinavica B* 88, 207–218.

KOSUNEN, T. U., DANIELSSON, D. & KJELLANDER, J. 1982 Serology of *Campylobacter fetus ss jejuni*. Serotyping of live bacteria by slide latex and co-agglutination tests. *Acta Pathologica, Microbiologica et Immunologica Scandinavica B* 90, 191–196.

LASTOVICA, A. J., MARSHALL, R. B. & PENNER, J. L. 1986 Campylobacter serotyping on shipped antigen extracts. *Lancet* i, 340.

LAUWERS, S., VAN ETTERIJCK, R & BOKKENHEUSER, V. D. 1985 Selective killing of *Campylobacter jejuni* and *C. coli* in the detection of infections with more than one serotype. In *Campylobacter III* eds. Pearson, A. D., Skirrow, M. B., Lior, H. & Rowe, B. pp. 67–69. London: Public Health Laboratory Service.

LAUWERS, S., VLAES, L. & BUTZLER, J. P. 1981 Campylobacter serotyping and epidemiology. *Lancet* i, 158–159.

LEY, A. B., HARRIS, J. P., BRINKLEY, M., LILES, B., JACK, J. A. & CAHAN, A. 1958 Circulating antibody directed against penicillin. *Science* 127, 1118–1119.

LIOR, H., WOODLANDS, D. L., EDGAR, J. A., LAROCHE, L. J. & GILL, P. 1982 Serotyping of *Campylobacter jejuni* by slide agglutination based on heat-labile antigenic factors. *Journal of Clinical Microbiology* 15, 761—768.

MANDAL, B. K., DE MOL, P. & BUTZLER, J. P. 1984 Clinical aspects of *Campylobacter* infections in humans. In *Campylobacter Infection in Man and Animals* ed. Butzler, J. P. pp. 21–31. Florida: CRC Press.

MILLS, S. D., BRADBURY, W. C. & PENNER, J. L. 1985 Basis for serological heterogeneity of thermostable antigens of *Campylobacter jejuni. Infection and Immunity* 50, 284–291.

MORRIS, J. A. & PARK, R. W. A. 1971 The isolation of microaerophilic vibrios. In *Isolation of Anaerobes* Society for Applied Bacteriology Technical Series No 5. ed. Shapton, D. A. & Board, R. G. pp. 207–217. London: Academic Press.

NAESS, V. & HOFSTAD, T. 1984a Chemical composition and biological activity of lipopolysaccharide prepared from type strains of *Campylobacter jejuni* and *Campylobacter coli*. *Acta Pathologica Microbiologica et Immunologica Scandinavica B* **92**, 217–222.

NAESS, V. & HOFSTAD, T. 1984b Chemical studies of partially hydrolysed lipopolysaccharides from four strains of *Campylobacter jejuni* and two strains of *Campylobacter coli*. *Journal of General Microbiology* **130**, 2783–2789.

NETER, E., BERTRAM, L. F., ZAK, D. A., MURDOCK, M. R. & ABESMAN, C. E. 1952 Studies on haemagglutination and hemolysis by *Escherichia coli* antisera. *Journal of Experimental Medicine* **96**, 1–15.

PATTON, C. M., BARRETT, T. J. & MORRIS, G. K. 1983 Serotyping *Campylobacter jejuni/coli* by two systems: the CDC experience. In: *Campylobacter II* eds. Pearson, A. D., Skirrow, M. B., Rowe, B., Davies, J. R. & Jones, D. M. London: Public Health Laboratory Service.

PENNER, J. L. & HENNESSY, J. N. 1980 Passive haemagglutination technique for serotyping *Campylobacter fetus* subsp. *jejuni* on the basis of heat-stable antigens. *Journal of Clinical Microbiology* **12**, 732–737.

RIGBY, C. E. 1984 Enzyme-linked immunosorbent assay for detection of *Salmonella* lipopolysaccharide in poultry specimens. *Applied and Environmental Microbiology* **47**, 1327–1330.

ROGOL, M., SECHTER, I., BRAUNSTEIN, I. & GERICHTER, C. B. 1982 Provisional antigenic scheme for *Campylobacter jejuni*. In *Campylobacter: Epidemiology, Pathogenesis and Biochemistry* ed. Newell, D. G. Lancaster: MTP Press.

SKIRROW, M. B., BENJAMIN, J., RAZI, M. H. H. & WATERMAN, S. 1982 Isolation, cultivation, and identification of *Campylobacter jejuni* and *C. coli*. In *Isolation and Identification Methods for Food Poisoning Organisms* Society for Applied Bacteriology Technical Series No 17. eds. Corry, J. E. L., Roberts, D. & Skinner, F. A. pp. 313–328. London: Academic Press.

WALKER, R. I., CALDWELL, M. B., LEE, E. C., GUERRY, P., TRUST, T. J. & RUIZ-PALACIOS, G. M. 1986 Pathophysiology of *Campylobacter* enteritis. *Microbiological Reviews* **50**, 81–94.

WONG, K. H., SKELTON, S. K., PATTON, C. M., FEELEY, J. C. & MORRIS, G. 1985 Typing of heat-stable and heat-labile antigens of *Campylobacter jejuni* and *Campylobacter coli* by coagglutination. *Journal of Clinical Microbiology* **21**, 702–707.

Emit Homogeneous Enzyme Immunoassay: Past, Present and Future

ANDY ANDERSON

Syva U.K., St. Ives House, Maidenhead, Berks SL6 1QS

Introduction

The introduction of the Emit Homogeneous Enzyme Immunoassay system for monitoring of aminoglycoside antibiotics revolutionised therapeutic drug monitoring of these substances. The Emit system allowed rapid accurate measurement of serum gentamicin levels and has now replaced bio-assay as the most popular technique for gentamicin measurement in the U.K.

The purpose of this chapter is to explain how the Emit system works and to look at its current use, the future developments of the system, and immunoassays in general.

The clinical advantages of a rapid aminoglycoside assay service are now well established. The use of Emit and other immunoassay systems for gentamicin monitoring has increased rapidly over the last few years. The main clinical advantages of a rapid assay are as follows: first, the clinician has more confidence to prescribe a dose at a level which will be sure to kill any bacteria that are present, measured by the peak concentration of the drug: secondly, the prevention of any side effects. Measuring the trough level of the drug guards against any failure of the patient to clear the antibiotic and thereby induce toxic side effects. The clinician can now have all the information he needs to make dosage adjustments before the next dose is given, whereas with the use of bio-assay, which was the most common analytical technique before the introduction of the immunoassays, the result was very often not available until after the next dose had been given to the patient.

The Principles of Immunoassays and, in Particular, Emit

Most immunoassays rely upon the concept of competition for specific antibody sites between a labelled antigen and antigen from the patient's serum. The first stage in any immunoassay is to produce the specific antibody for the drug to be measured.

Immunological Techniques
in Microbiology

The procedure for this is shown in Fig. 1. Substances of low molecular weight, e.g. most drugs, will not generally elicit an immune response in an animal. Specific antibodies to drugs are thus made by attaching the compound to be assayed to a protein carrier—most commonly bovine serum albumin—to produce a larger antigen. Animals are immunized with this new antigen and, after several months, the antibody-bearing gamma globulin fraction of the animal's blood is isolated. The possible binding sites in the antibodies indicated in Fig. 1 are represented by the two half circles. An antibody will bind the specific shape of the molecule for which it is designed leaving unbound the variety of other biochemical components present in the sample.

The second stage is to choose and produce the biochemical label which will determine the concentration of antigen in the patient's serum. The Emit system is a homogeneous enzyme immunoassay, the word *homogeneous* indicating that no step is needed, as in many other immunoassays, to separate antibody-bound from unbound labelled antigen. The unique component of the Emit assay is the enzyme labelled drug, the production of which is shown in Fig. 2. The choice of enzyme label varies from assay to assay in the Emit system and depends upon several criteria.

1 It should possess a high specific activity at a pH that does not impair antigen-antibody binding.

2 It should be readily available in highly purified soluble and stable form at reasonable cost.

3 It should be simply and very sensitively detectable and should be absent from biological fluids.

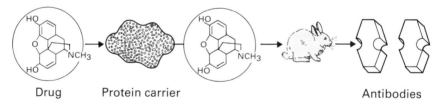

Drug   Protein carrier   Antibodies

FIG. 1. Antibody preparation.

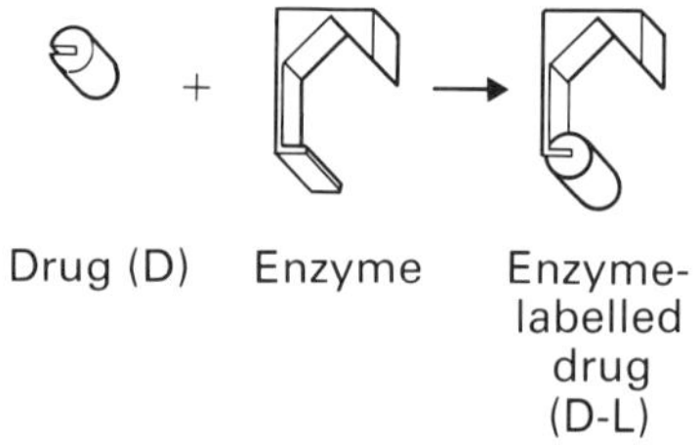

Drug (D)   Enzyme   Enzyme-
                    labelled
                    drug
                    (D-L)

FIG. 2. Enzyme-labelled drug production.

4 It should also not be inhibited by substances present in biological fluids and should possess reactive groups throughout which can be linked to other molecules without significantly impairing either the enzyme activity or the antigen/antibody binding.

The enzyme chosen for the Emit gentamicin assay was glucose-6-phosphate dehydrogenase. This enzyme is attached to gentamicin molecules to produce the enzyme labelled drug as shown in Fig. 2.

With the antibody and enzyme labelled drug in hand, we now have the two key components for the Emit immunoassay system. Figure 3 illustrates the Emit principle for a typical gentamicin assay. The substrate for the enzyme glucose-6-phosphate (G6P) and the co-factor for the enzyme, nicotinamide adenine dinucleotide (NAD), are contained together with the antibodies to gentamicin in

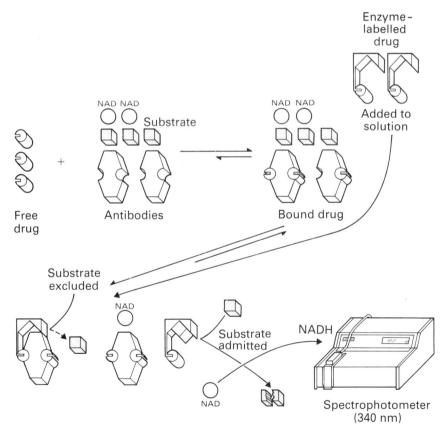

FIG. 3.   Emit principle.

what is known as Reagent A. Reagent B consists of the enzyme-labelled drug. The addition of the patient's serum to a mixture of Reagent A and B causes the reaction seen in Fig. 3. The drug in the patient's serum and the enzyme labelled drug compete for antibody binding sites. The more drug from the patient's serum the more enzyme labelled drug will be free in solution and able to act on substrate. There is, therefore, a direct correlation between the amount of drug in the patient's serum and enzyme activity.

The system provides an intrinsic amplification since one molecule of gentamicin in the sample frees one molecule of enzyme-labelled gentamicin which in turn catalyses the conversion of many molecules of the substrate to product. The unique homogeneity of the Emit system is the result of the steric hindrance of the enzyme when attached to the antibody, thus preventing enzyme-substrate reaction and thereby removing the need for a separation step.

The Emit assay procedure is simple and reaction times are quite short due to the high specific activity of the enzyme label and antibodies and to the biochemical amplification feature.

The kinetic determination of enzyme activity requires 30 s and a single assay is complete in 1 min. Drug analysis can be made within several minutes of sample receipt using the appropriate instrumentation. Reagents are supplied in 100-assay kits and include Reagents A and B, a specific buffer for the assay, together with calibrators covering the normal range of gentamicin concentration of 0–16 µg/ml. The Emit assay can be performed on many different types of instruments including various types of spectrophotometers and centrifugal analysers. The instrument system most commonly used in the U.K. microbiology laboratories, however, is supplied by Syva specifically for use with its Emit assays. The system consists of a pipetter diluter which is used to take up the sample of 50 µl and add to it specific quantities of Reagent A and B as well as the buffer necessary for the reaction. Two 1-in-6 dilutions are made by this diluter into specific analytical cups and, once Reagent B has been added to the final mixture, this is then aspirated into the spectrophotometer supplied with the system. This spectrophotometer has a micro flowthrough cuvette, the temperature of which is specifically and tightly controlled at 30 °C, the optimum temperature for the enzyme reaction to take place.

The amount of the product, NADH (Fig. 3), is directly proportional to the amount of drug in the patient's serum. NADH absorbs light at 340 nm and the spectrophotometer is set up to read the reaction at this wavelength. The absorbance increases as NADH is produced and the rate at which this product is produced over a 30 s time period is measured by the computer supplied with the system. This rate of reaction increases according to the amount of gentamicin present in the patient's serum. The computer plots this and correlates the rate of reaction against previously entered standard curves to quantitate the antibiotic in the patient's serum.

Emit assays are therefore rapid and simple to perform and, as it is a homogeneous method, it requires no separation stage. No sample preparation or extraction is necessary and reagents are safe and show a good long-term stability. Assays can be performed on simple laboratory equipment and sample requirements are small, lending the method to paediatric testing.

All immunoassays have one major limitation: they are single analyte or family analyte methods in contrast to high resolution chromatographic techniques. Likewise their use in exploratory analytical work is limited. The methods are, however, extremely useful in routine analytical determinations that require both senstivity and specificity. Emit assays are available for gentamicin, tobramycin, amikacin and netilmicin as well as many other therapeutic drugs.

Future Developments

A drawback of the Emit system has been that reagents are supplied in lyophilized form and reconstituted in the laboratory by the addition of distilled water. Once in this reconstituted form they have a stability of 3 months. Due to the changes in the activities of NAD and antibodies over time, the laboratories have been required to check and re-enter standard curves on a regular basis over this 3 month period. Thus laboratories with small workloads do not find Emit in this form cost-effective due to the fact that they do not use a full kit within the stated 3 month stability period. Even laboratories with relatively high workloads use a proportion of their reagent on entering calibration curves into the instrument.

Syva have adapted the Emit technique to overcome both these problems. The new system is called Quantitative Single Test or QST and involves two major developments. The first is the development of a dry powder filling system which has enabled single vials to be produced containing enough Reagent A, B and buffer in lyophilized form for a single assay. The reagent remains lyophilized until the moment of its use, thus giving exceptionally long stability of 18 months or more to each individual test. This not only allows for small workloads to be performed without kits having to be thrown away but also leads to an extended standard curve stability as reagents are not in liquid form and thus do not deteriorate.

The QST instrument has been developed to handle these vials and is one of the most simple methods now available for performing gentamicin or aminoglycoside monitoring. To perform an assay, the operator simply unscrews the vial and places it in the instrument, which contains a heater that heats the vial to the optimum 30 °C. By pressing a single button a specific volume of patient's serum is drawn up into the vial and from then on the procedure is totally automatic. The instrument adds water to reconstitute the reagent, the vortex mixes the reagent and passes it into the spectrophotometer where the normal Emit reaction takes place. The QST system therefore provides laboratories with an even more simple and accurate method of gentamicin assay and allows them to offer an assay service on all aminoglycosides even if they are only used rarely, without the cost penalty of having unused reagent thrown away.

There are several other immunoassays available for aminoglycoside monitoring, including fluorescence polarization immunoassay, substrate labelled fluorescence immunoassay and assays utilizing chemiluminesence.

Future developments in the field will include further refinements of these systems to make even simpler and more cost-effective assays available, together with new assays for antibiotics such as chloramphenical and vancomycin.

Further in the future it should be possible to perform assays at the patient's bedside rather than having to send specimens off to the laboratory. The first system available for such assays is already marketed by Syva U.K. and is called AccuLevel™ and is at the moment available only for the antiasthmatic drug theophylline. The system requires no instrumentation, can be performed on a finger prick sample, i.e. whole blood, and is as accurate as a normal immunoassay. It is only a matter of time before this type of technology enables gentamicin and aminoglycoside levels to be determined when and where they are required.

Enzyme Linked Immunosorbent Assays for the Detection of *Salmonella* in Foods

JULIE A. CLAYDEN, SUSAN J. ALCOCK AND M. F. STRINGER

Microbiology Department, Campden Food Preservation Research Association, Chipping Campden, Gloucestershire GL55 6LD

Introduction

Salmonella infections accounted for 13 201 (86%) of the total number of 15 312 food poisoning cases reported in England and Wales in 1984 (Anon., 1986). Many European countries also reported a high percentage of cases of salmonellosis, for example, in 1982, Belgium 86.3%; Federal Republic of Germany 71%; the Netherlands 77% and Scotland 79.2% (WHO, 1982). In the same year *Salmonella* was the most frequently isolated bacterial pathogen in the U.S.A., causing 18.6% of the total number of 11 050 confirmed cases of foodborne disease (MMWR, 1986).

Although the annual statistics relating to the incidence of food poisoning outbreaks show fluctuation, the occurrence of *Salmonella*-related outbreaks has increased dramatically since the mid 1960s, the predominant serotype being *S. typhimurium*. Furthermore, epidemiological studies of *Salmonella* food poisoning have indicated that outbreaks associated with low numbers are increasingly prevalent (Blaser & Newman, 1982; Gill *et al.*, 1983 and D'Aoust *et al.*, 1985).

Traditional cultural methods using enrichment and selective media for the detection of *Salmonella* require up to 7 days to produce confirmed postive results (AOAC, 1984; ISO, 1981). Increasing economic pressures are strengthening the need to shorten the holding times before foods are positively cleared for *Salmonella*. There is, therefore, a need for methods which are cheaper, simpler and more rapid than existing cultural procedures.

Many of the alternative methods involve the use of labelled antibodies which are specific to *Salmonella*. The most recent of these immunological procedures is the Enzyme Linked Immunosorbent Assay (ELISA). The first ELISA developed for the detection of *Salmonella* in foods used cells spotted and fixed onto cellulose acetate membrane filters (Krysinski & Heimsch, 1977). This was not satisfactory because the antibodies used were impure, and in 1978 Minnich improved this procedure by using purified polyvalent antisera. Other methods using polyclonal-H antiserum have been reported (Swaminathan & Ayres, 1980; Minnich *et al.*, 1982;

Immunological Techniques
in Microbiology

Aleixo *et al.*, 1984, and Anderson & Hartman, 1985) and, although the IgG fraction has been purified to eliminate the IgM component, the amount of cross-reactivity of the antibody preparations in these methods was still considered a problem (Mattingly *et al.*, 1985).

An ELISA using a monoclonal antibody (MOPC 467, from an IgA myeloma) to detect *Salmonella* was first reported by Robison *et al.* (1983), but the technique only detected 94% of the serotypes examined. This problem was overcome by the addition of a second monoclonal antibody hybridoma referred to as 6H4 (Mattingly, 1984). Mattingly & Gehle (1984) substituted horseradish peroxidase for alkaline phosphatase, and introduced a degree of automation by using polycarbonate coated metal beads, thus eliminating the antibody/microtitre plate coupling step from the assay.

Research in *Salmonella* ELISA techniques has resulted in commercially available kits for the detection of the organism in foods. The two kits currently available in the U.K. are the Bio-Enzabead *Salmonella* screen kit (Organon Teknika Corp., Durham, U.S.A.) and the Bactelisa screening kit for *Salmonella* (Kirkegaard and Perry Laboratories, Maryland, U.S.A.). The Bio-Enzabead kit utilizes the two monoclonals developed by Robison *et al.* (1983) and Mattingly (1984), whilst the Bactelisa kit supplies a polyclonal antibody preparation specific to *Salmonella*. The antibodies are bound to a bead (Bio-Enzabead) or a well in a microtitre plate (Bactelisa).

In each method the sample is added and any *Salmonella* cells present bind to the immobilized antibodies. Enzyme labelled antibodies are added and these attach to the bound *Salmonella* cells. An appropriate substrate is introduced and the bound enzyme acts on this to form a coloured end-product, the intensity of which can be read by using a plate reader.

In the present study, both commercial kits were evaluated for their ability to detect *Salmonella* in artificially inoculated frozen slurries of raw meat. The results were compared with those obtained by using two established conventional cultural procedures. The sensitivity of each method was tested using a range of inoculation levels. The methods were also compared for their ability to detect a range of *Salmonella* serotypes.

Methods and Materials

Bacterial cultures

The *Salmonella* cultures used are listed below; those coded BR, SSU and CCC were obtained from Public Health Laboratory Service, Colindale, London; Centres for Disease Control (CDC), Atlanta, Georgia, U.S.A. and Colworth Culture Collection, Unilever Limited, Sharnbrook, Bedfordshire respectively: *S. agona* BR 1786, *S. anatum* NCTC 5779, *S. bredeney* NCTC 5731, *S. eastbourne* SSU 3183, *S. enteritidis* NCTC 4444, *S. hadar* NCTC 9877, *S. heidelberg* SSU SO1S/E363, *S. indiana*

NCTC 11304, *S. infantis* NCTC 10679, *S. montevideo* NCTC 5747, *S. napoli* BR 3427, *S. newport* SSU 3724, *S. panama* NCTC 5774, *S. saint paul* NCTC 6022, *S. senftenberg* NCTC 4969, *S. senftenberg* NCTC 9959, *S. stanley* NCTC 92, *S. typhimurium* NCTC 74, *S. typhimurium* phage type 10 CCC166 STM 10, *S. typhimurium* phage type 12 CCC167 STM 12 and *S. virchow* NCTC 5742.

Food substrates

Raw whole chickens and beef steak, obtained from a local butcher, were immersed in a 50 ppm solution of sodium hypochlorite for 10 min to remove surface contamination, and then thoroughly rinsed to remove excess hypochlorite. Excess fat was removed from the beef and the meat was cut into approximately 2 cm cubes. The chickens were skinned and jointed, and the flesh was removed from the bones; for both beef and chicken the meat was slurried using a Fryma colloidal mill (Aheinfelven, Switzerland). Portions, 250 g, were weighed into stomacher bags (Seward Medical Supplies, London), flattened to remove excess air, heat sealed and blast-frozen to −18 °C. The slurries were checked for the absence of *Salmonella* using the cultural methods chosen for the evaluation, and a total viable count was determined (Hall, 1982).

Slurry inoculation

The chicken and beef slurries were thawed overnight at ambient temperature, inoculated with stationary phase *Salmonella* cultures grown in nutrient broth (Oxoid CM1) at 30 °C for 3 days. Slurries were then homogenized for 3 min using a Colworth stomacher (A. J. Seward, London). Bags containing the samples were flattened by hand, heat sealed, blast-frozen to −18 °C and held in frozen storage at −19 ± 1 °C for 1 month. Some of these packs were subsequently used as uninoculated controls.

Experiment 1 : detection of S. typhimurium

The Association of Official Analytical Chemists (AOAC), Hall's and Bio-Enzabead methods were compared. *Salmonella typhimurium* NCTC 74 was inoculated into chicken and beef slurries such that after freezing and thawing (which results in about one log cycle decrease in viable cells), there were three samples each with approximate levels of 1.0 and 10.0 viable *Salmonella* cells/g of food, and six samples with a level of 0.1 cells/g of food.

Experiment 2 : detection of Salmonella serotypes

The AOAC, Hall's methods and both ELISA kits were compared for their ability to detect 21 *Salmonella* serotypes. Chicken and beef slurries were artificially

inoculated with *S. agona, S. anatum, S. bredeney, S. eastbourne, S. enteritidis, S. hadar,*
S. heidelberg, S. indiana, S. infantis, S. montevideo, S. napoli, S. newport, S. panama, S.
saint paul, S. senftenberg NCTC 4969, *S. senftenberg* NCTC 9959, *S. stanley, S.*
typhimurium NCTC 74, *S. typhimurium* phage type 10, *S. typhimurium* phage type 12
and *S. virchow.* One sample of each slurry was incoculated with one serotype such
that post-frozen storage levels of 0.1 and 1.0 cells/g of food were attained.

Culture methods

The two cultural procedures used for the comparison with the two ELISA methods
were those of the AOAC (1984), and Hall (1982). The AOAC method involved a
pre-enrichment step in lactose broth followed by selective enrichments in
tetrathionate and selenite-cystine broths. Loopfuls of the selective broths were
streaked onto selective plates of xylose lysine desoxycholate agar, hektoen enteric
agar and bismuth sulphite agar, from which presumptive colonies were inoculated
onto slants of triple sugar iron agar, lysine iron agar and finally into urea broth. The
incubation times, temperatures and media composition were according to the
AOAC method.

Hall's procedure involved a resuscitation period in peptone buffered diluent
followed by selective enrichments in tetrationate (Oxoid CM29) and selenite (Oxoid
CM395) broths. Loopfuls of these broths were then streaked onto selective plates of
desoxycholate citrate lysine sucrose agar (DCLSA, Oxoid CM393) and brilliant
green agar (BGA, Oxoid CM263). Presumptive colonies were inoculated into
Kohn's two tube medium (Kohn No. 1, Oxoid CM179 and Kohn No. 2, Oxoid
CM181) and lysine broth. The incubation times and temperatures used were those
described in Hall's method.

ELISA techniques

Both kits contained all the specific reagents necessary to perform the assays,
although with the Bactelisa test distilled water and immunoassay plates were not
provided.

With the Bio-Enzabead assay slurries were pre- and selectively enriched
according to the AOAC (1984) procedure: 0.5 ml of each selective broth was
inoculated into one tube containing 10 ml M-broth (Difco 0940-01-2) and
incubated at 35 °C for 6 h. Ten millilitres of this selective broth were removed and
centrifuged at 1000 g for 20 min in a swingout head centrifuge (Denley Instruments
Limited, Bolney, England). The residual M-broth was stored at 4 °C for confirmatory
tests. Following the centrifugation step, the supernatant was discarded and the
pellet was resuspended in 1 ml peptone buffered saline, vortex mixed and heat
treated in a boiling water bath for 20 min. These samples were held overnight at
room temperature (approximately 25 °C) prior to the ELISA.

The Bio-Enzabead assay was started by dispensing 0.2 ml of the control or test samples into a 96 well microtitre plate. A single antibody-coated bead was added to each well except for the substrate blank well, and the plate was then incubated at 37 °C for 20 min with agitation at about 100 rpm in a shaking plate incubator (Organon Teknika Corp.). The beads were transferred between plates of reagents by the use of a magnetic transfer device (Organon Teknika Corp.). The beads were washed in wash solution (wash 1) by raising and lowering the beads 12 times into a microtitre plate containing 0.3 ml of the wash reagent per well. Conjugate, 0.2 ml, was dispensed into the wells of another microtitre plate. The beads were transferred into this plate and incubated for 20 min at 37 °C with agitation. After the conjugate incubation, the beads were washed as previously described by raising and lowering in wash 1 three times and then nine times in wash 2, to remove unbound conjugate. The beads were then added to 0.2 ml substrate and incubated for 10 min at room temperature without agitation, after which 0.025 ml of the reagent which stops the enzyme reaction was added to each well and the plate was swirled gently by hand to disperse the colour before removing the beads. The optical density (OD) of the contents of the wells was measured by using a plate reader (Organon Teknika Corp.) at 405 nm. The substrate blank well was used to zero the plate reader. For a valid test, the average OD of the two negative controls should read < 0.12 and the positive control > 0.2. Samples reading ⩾ 0.2 are then scored as positive for *Salmonella*.

Pre- and selective enrichment steps for the Bactelisa technique also followed the AOAC (1984) procedure. With the Bactelisa method, 0.1 ml of the pre-enrichment broth was inoculated into 10 ml each of the selective broths and a 2 ml sample was removed from each. These samples (labelled 'IN') were heat treated in a boiling water bath for 15 min and then stored at 4 °C overnight, whilst the remaining selective broths were incubated at 35 °C. After incubation a 2 ml sample (labelled 'OUT') was removed from each selective broth and heat treated as before. All samples were allowed to reach room temperature prior to the ELISA.

The Bactelisa procedure was initiated by adding 0.1 ml capture antibody solution to the appropriate wells of a 96 well microtitre plate (Dynatech, M129B Dynatech Laboratories Ltd., Billingshurst, Sussex). After incubation at room temperature for 60 min the plate was emptied by rapid inversion and 0.3 ml of 1x bacterial diluent/blocking solution was added to each well. The reaction was allowed to proceed for 10 min and the plate then emptied. On all occasions the residual fluid was removed by tapping the plate on a paper towel. Next, 0.1 ml of the controls (two each of positive controls, selective broths and bacterial diluent/blocking solution) or heat-treated samples were added and incubated for 60 min at room temperature. The plate was then emptied and washed twice. For the wash procedure each well was filled with wash solution and the plate was emptied. Enzyme labelled antibody solution (0.1 ml) was then added to each well and incubated for 60 min at room temperature. The plate was emptied, washed three times and given a 5 min soak with the wash solution. The plate was emptied, thoroughly tapped and 0.1 ml enzyme substrate solution was dispensed into each well.

After sufficient colour development (10–15 min was found to be optimal) the plate was read visually or with a plate reader (Dynatech Laboratories Ltd.). For a valid test the positive control should be a dark green colour, the bacterial diluent/ blocking solution colourless and the selective broths faintly green. Any sample where the colour of the 'OUT' sample was observed to be a darker green than that of the 'IN' was considered to be positive for viable *Salmonella*. No guidelines on the interpretation of OD values were supplied with the Bactelisa kit. Therefore, an 'OUT' OD value of greater than 150% that of the 'IN' OD reading was chosen as a positive viable *Salmonella* result.

For the purposes of this study, ELISA results were confirmed by plating loopfuls of selected samples of the M-broth (Bio-Enzabead) and selective broths (Bactelisa) onto selective agars, and through the confirmatory tests described in the AOAC method.

Results

The results obtained are summarized in Tables 1–3 as *Salmonella* presence or absence in the slurries as determined by each method.

Experiment 1. detection of S. typhimurium

The AOAC and Bio-Enzabead ELISA methods both detected *Salmonella* in all of the beef samples to which *S. typhimurium* had been added at each of the three inoculation levels of 10, 1.0 and 0.1 cells/g. By Hall's method, *Salmonella* could only be detected in seven of the 12 inoculated samples (Table 1). *Salmonella* was detected in the majority of the inoculated chicken samples by both the AOAC and Hall's cultural methods, whereas the Bio-Enzabead system yielded more negative than positive results, and there was no correlation with the level of inoculation. In this experiment the three methods all gave *Salmonella* negative results for the uninoculated chicken, but positive results for the uninoculated beef controls, which indicates that the beef controls were naturally contaminated with *Salmonella*.

Experiment 2. detection of Salmonella serotypes

The detection by the two cultural and the two ELISA methods of 21 *Salmonella* serotypes individually inoculated into chicken and beef slurries is compared in Tables 2 and 3. The AOAC method produced positive results for *Salmonella* in all of the artificially contaminated chicken slurries. With this method positive results were also obtained for all inoculated beef samples except for two serotypes.

TABLE 1. *Detection of* S. typhimurium *NCTC 74, in frozen inoculated chicken and beef slurries*

Food substrate	Inoculation level (cells/g of food)	Sample number	Hall	AOAC	Bio-Enzabead ELISA
Beef	0	1	+	+	+
	0.1	1	+	+	+
		2	+	+	+
		3	+	+	+
		4	+	+	+
		5	+	+	+
		6	−	+	+
	1.0	1	−	+	+
		2	−	+	+
		3	−	+	+
	10.0	1	+	+	+
		2	−	+	+
		3	+	+	+
Chicken	0	1	−	−	−
	0.1	1	−	+	−
		2	+	+	−
		3	+	+	+
		4	+	+	+
		5	+	+	−
		6	+	+	−
	1.0	1	+	−	−
		2	+	+	+
		3	+	+	−
	10.0	1	+	+	−
		2	+	+	+
		3	+	+	−

The Bio-Enzabead kit detected *Salmonella* in all but one of the inoculated chicken and beef samples. Confirmatory tests on selected samples verified the ELISA results although four samples were shown to be *Salmonella* negative.

In the first run the Bactelisa colour changes were distinct and were assessed visually whilst in the second run some colour differences were difficult to distinguish and therefore, in addition, the plates were read with a plate reader. *Salmonella* positive results were obtained for all but one of the inoculated beef and chicken samples in run 1, and these were subsequently confirmed by cultural methods (Table 2). In run 2 the inoculated samples were all *Salmonella* positive using the plate reader although eight of them were negative when the plate was assessed visually. It was sometimes difficult to correlate the results assessed either by eye or using the plate reader to the results obtained by subsequent cultural confirmations (Table 3).

TABLE 2. *Detection of Salmonella serotypes in inoculated frozen chicken and beef slurries (run 1)*

Salmonella serotype	Inoculation level (cells/g)	Beef						Chicken					
		AOAC	Hall	Bio-Enzabead ELISA result	confirm	Bactelisa ELISA result	confirm*	AOAC	Hall	Bio-Enzabead ELISA result	confirm	Bactelisa ELISA result	confirm*
Uninoculated control	0	+	−	+	NT	−	+	−	−	−	NT	−	−
stanley	0.1	+	−	+	+	+	+	+	+	+	+	+	+
	1.0	+	+	+	+	+	+	+	+	+	+	+	+
agona	0.1	+	+	+	+	+	+	+	+	+	+	+	+
	1.0	+	+	+	+	+	+	+	+	+	+	+	+
hadar	0.1	+	+	+	NT	+	+	+	+	+	NT	+	+
	1.0	+	+	+	NT	+	+	+	+	+	NT	+	−
enteritidis	0.1	+	+	+	+	+	+	+	+	+	+	+	+
	1.0	+	+	+	+	+	+	+	+	+	+	+	+
typhimurium 10	0.1	+	−	+	+	+	+	+	+	+	+	+	+
	1.0	+	+	+	+	+	+	+	+	+	+	+	+
typhimurium 12	0.1	+	+	+	NT	+	+	+	+	+	NT	+	+
	1.0	+	+	+	NT	+	+	+	+	+	NT	+	+
bredeney	0.1	+	−	+	+	−	+	+	+	+	+	+	+
	1.0	+	−	+	+	+	+	+	+	+	+	+	+
senftenberg 4969	0.1	+	+	+	NT	+	+	+	−	+	NT	+	+
	1.0	+	+	+	NT	+	+	+	+	+	NT	+	+
senftenberg 9959	0.1	+	−	+	+	+	+	+	+	+	+	+	+
	1.0	+	+	+	+	+	+	+	+	+	+	+	+
infantis	0.1	+	+	+	NT	+	+	+	−	+	NT	+	+
	1.0	+	+	+	NT	+	+	+	+	+	NT	+	+
virchow	0.1	+	+	+	NT	+	+	+	−	+	NT	+	+
	1.0	+	+	+	NT	+	+	+	+	+	NT	+	+

* Assessed visually. NT = not tested.

TABLE 3. *Detection of Salmonella serotypes in inoculated frozen chicken and beef slurries (run 2)*

Salmonella serotype	Inoculation level (cells/g)	Beef AOAC	Beef Hall	Beef Bio-Enzabead ELISA result	Beef Bio-Enzabead ELISA confirm	Beef Bactelisa ELISA result†*	Beef Bactelisa ELISA confirm	Chicken AOAC	Chicken Hall	Chicken Bio-Enzabead ELISA result	Chicken Bio-Enzabead ELISA confirm	Chicken Bactelisa ELISA result*	Chicken Bactelisa ELISA confirm
Uninoculated control	0	−	−	−	NT	+ −	−	+	+	+	−	+ −	+
	0	−	−	−	NT	+ −	NT	−	−	−	NT	+ −	−
	0	−	−	−	NT	+ −	−	−	−	−	NT	+ −	−
anatum	0.1	+	−	+	NT	+ −	+	+	−	+	NT	+ +	NT
	1.0	+	−	+	NT	+ −	+	+	+	+	NT	+ +	NT
eastbourne	0.1	+	+	+	NT	+ +	NT	+	+	+	NT	+ +	NT
	1.0	+	+	+	NT	+ +	NT	+	−	+	NT	+ +	NT
heidelberg	0.1	+	+	+	NT	+ +	NT	+	+	+	NT	+ +	NT
	1.0	+	+	+	NT	+ +	−	+	−	+	NT	+ +	NT
indiana	0.1	−	−	+	NT	+ +	−	+	−	+	NT	+ +	NT
	1.0	−	−	+	NT	+ −	+	+	−	+	NT	+ +	−
montevideo	0.1	+	+	+	NT	+ +	NT	+	+	+	NT	+ +	NT
	1.0	+	+	+	NT	+ +	NT	+	+	+	NT	+ +	NT
napoli	0.1	+	−	+	NT	+ +	NT	+	−	+	NT	+ +	NT
	1.0	+	−	+	NT	+ +	NT	+	−	+	NT	+ +	NT
newport	0.1	+	+	+	NT	+ +	+	+	+	+	NT	+ +	NT
	1.0	+	+	+	NT	+ +	NT	+	−	+	NT	+ +	NT
panama	0.1	+	+	+	NT	+ +	NT	+	+	+	−	+ +	−
	1.0	+	+	+	NT	+ +	NT	+	+	+	NT	+ +	NT
saint paul	0.1	+	+	+	NT	+ +	−	+	+	+	NT	+ +	NT
	1.0	+	+	+	NT	+ +	−	+	+	+	NT	+ +	NT
typhimurium 74	0.1	−	−	+	−	+ −	−	+	+	−	−	+ −	−
	1.0	−	−	+	+	+ +	−	+	−	−	−	+	−

* Assessed visually. † Assessed using plate reader. NT = not tested.

Hall's method failed to detect *Salmonella* in three beef and four chicken samples at the 0.1 cell/g level, one chicken sample at 1.0 cell/g and two beef samples at both levels. Moreover, three serotypes were not detected in either chicken or beef at any inoculation level.

The uninoculated controls for the first run of the experiment (Table 2) proved negative for *Salmonella* by all methods for the chicken sample but some test results were positive for beef. The controls for the run 2 serotypes were all *Salmonella* negative for the beef samples, except by the Bactelisa kit where the results were obtained by means of a plate reader (Table 3). Similar results were recorded for the uninoculated chicken controls except for one sample which was *Salmonella* positive by three out of the four methods.

Discussion

Ninety five per cent of the chicken and 90.5% of the beef slurry samples artificially inoculated with *Salmonella* and frozen at levels of 0.1 and 1.0 cells/g in Experiment 2 were positive for *Salmonella* by both the Bio-Enzabead ELISA and AOAC cultural methods. However, 9.5% of the beef samples were positive by the Bio-Enzabead kit alone, whilst *Salmonella* was detected in 5% of the chicken samples by the AOAC method and not by the others. The artificially inoculated slurry samples positive by the cultural method alone suggest that false-negative results were produced by the Bio-Enzabead kit. These slurry samples, however, had been inoculated with *S. typhimurium* (NCTC 74) which is thought to have undergone changes during long-term storage.

In a study of 120 food samples naturally contaminated with *Salmonella*, Todd *et al.* (1986) detected the organism in 58% of the samples by both the Bio-Enzabead ELISA method and the ISO standard cultural procedure. However, 18% and 1.7% of the samples were positive by only the Bio-Enzabead kit and cultural methods respectively. They suggested that these results could be attributable to competing microbes.

D'Aoust & Sewell (1986) evaluated the Bio-Enzabead kit consisting of one monoclonal antibody, and obtained positive results for 96% of 28 naturally contaminated food samples, though 25% were later considered to be false-positives. These false-positive results were also attributed to the competing microflora, especially cross-reactivity with *Citrobacter*.

Competition of the inoculated *Salmonella* serotypes with the natural microbial flora of the beef and chicken slurries is thought to account for the *Salmonella* negative results obtained by the use of Hall's cultural method in Experiments 1 and 2. Presumptive *Salmonella* colonies were often observed on the edge of bacterial growth on the selective agars. Despite careful inoculation of these colonies into multiple confirmatory tests these presumptive salmonellae were often overgrown by other bacteria.

Although several workers have evaluated the Bio-Enzabead kit, there have been no publications relating to the Bactelisa kit. In Experiment 2, run 1, the AOAC and Bactelisa kit detected *Salmonella* in all of the chicken and 95% of the beef slurries. The results in run 1 were attained by visual assessment of the microtitre plates, and the colour differences of the 'IN' and 'OUT' samples were distinct. One of the disadvantages of the Bactelisa kit is that a 'STOP' solution is not added to terminate the enzyme/substrate reaction, and the kit instructions do not clearly indicate how long after the addition of the substrate the plates should be read. This can lead to excess colour production which increases the possibility of false readings.

One of the other major drawbacks with the Bactelisa kit is that guidance is not provided with the kit instructions as to the interpretation of OD values should the plate be assessed by using a plate reader. The user is left to decide the threshold values which determine whether a sample is *Salmonella* positive or negative. This not only allows for user error but introduces a degree of variation since the colour development is not limited. These points were illustrated with Experiment 2, run 2, where the colour difference of the 'IN' and 'OUT' samples was difficult to distinguish. All of the slurry samples were considered *Salmonella* positive by OD value interpretation, whereas only 75% of the beef and 85% of the chicken slurries were positive by visual assessment. This could suggest that either the interpretation of the OD values was erroneous or that the kit produced false negative results.

Although the slurries were examined for the absence of *Salmonella* prior to inoculation some samples were naturally contaminated with *Salmonella*. In an attempt to overcome the control contamination problems the number of uninoculated samples was increased from one to three per slurry in run 2.

The problem of uninoculated controls appearing *Salmonella* positive was discussed by Beckers *et al.* (1986). These workers evaluated the Bio-Enzabead kit, and using the guidance on OD value interpretation described in the kit instructions, they found all of their uninoculated minced meat samples to be *Salmonella* positive. Similarly, the OD values obtained for the negative controls supplied with the kit were above those accepted as a valid test (i.e. 0.12).

In this evaluation the OD values for the Bio-Enzabead controls were within the limits quoted in the instructions. The values for the inoculated slurry samples were, however, sometimes close to the recommended threshold value of 0.2 for a positive sample.

The Bio-Enzabead and Bactelisa kits have a minimal requirement of about 10^6 cells. Since *Salmonella* are often present in low numbers, the foods need to undergo both pre- and selective enrichments prior to assay. In contrast to the Bactelisa kit, the Bio-Enzabead kit in addition to pre- and selective enrichments also requires an elective enrichment in M-broth followed by centrifugation.

Both kits have a shelf life of 28 days once opened, and produce *Salmonella* positive or negative results in 3 days. In this evaluation, the cultural methods yielded negative results in 3 days but required a further 4 days to confirm *Salmonella* positive results. The instructions provided with both of the ELISA kits recommend that all *Salmonella* positive results be culturally confirmed.

The utilization of microtitre plates involves the use of small volumes of reagents, keeping the costs to a minimum. Not all of the plate need be used in one assay and the Bio-Enzabead food samples may be stored for up to 3 days until sufficient numbers are gathered to fill a microtitre plate.

The Bactelisa kit instructions recommend that two wells be designated to each 'IN' and 'OUT' sample. This results in 22 samples per plate compared to 96 with the Bio-Enzabead kit.

There are two possible areas of potential user error with the kits, the first being cross-contamination of antigens and reagents. Pipettors should always be held vertical, clean tips used and the greatest care taken to avoid carry-over of solutions. The wash procedures are the other potential source of error. Microtitre plate wells of the Bactelisa assay should always be throughly emptied. When using the Bio-Enzabead kit magnetic transfer device the user should ensure that the magnet is raised and lowered to its extreme positions, and that the plates are inserted correctly.

To conclude, the advantages and disadvantages of each *Salmonella* ELISA kit have been discussed, the relative merits of which must be ultimately dictated by the needs of the user. Whilst the Bio-Enzabead kit is more expensive and requires a larger initial capital outlay for equipment, it has gained AOAC approval and offers a comprehensive standardized method.

Acknowledgements

The authors wish to thank Barbara Robison and Marc Geens (Organon Teknika Corp.), Christopher Hall and Jill Horswill (Biokits Limited) and Jeanette West (Uniscience Limited) for kindly supplying the kits and equipment necessary for this evaluation.

References

ALEIXO, J. A. G., SWAMINATHAN, B. & MINNICH, S. A. 1984 *Salmonella* detection in foods and feeds in 27 hours by enzyme immunoassay. *The Journal of Microbiological Methods* 2, 135–145.

ANDERSON, J. M. & HARTMAN, P. A. 1985 Direct immunoassay for detection of salmonellae in foods and feeds. *Applied and Environmental Microbiology* 49, 1124–1127.

ANON. 1986 Foodborne disease surveillance in England and Wales 1984. *British Medical Journal* 293, 1424–1427.

ASSOCIATION OF OFFICIAL ANALYTICAL CHEMISTS (AOAC) 1984 *Official Methods of Analysis*. 14th Edn. pp. 663–971. Arlington, Virginia, U.S.A.: AOAC.

BECKERS, H. J., TIPS, P. D., DELFGOU-VAN ASCH, E. & PETERS, R. 1986 Evaluation of an enzyme immunoassay technique for the detection of salmonellas in minced beef. *Letters in Applied Microbiology* 2, 53–56.

BLASER, M. J. & NEWMAN, L. S. 1982 A review of human salmonellosis. I. Infective dose. *Reviews of Infectious Diseases* **4**, 1096–1106.

D'AOUST, J-Y. & SEWELL, A. M. 1986 Detection of *Salmonella* by the Enzyme Immunoassay (EIA) technique. *Journal of Food Science* **2**, 484–488, 507.

D'AOUST, J-Y., WARBURTON, D. W. & SEWELL, A. M. 1985 *Salmonella typhimurium* phage-type 10 from cheddar cheese implicated in a major Canadian foodborne outbreak. *Journal of Food Protection* **48**, 1062–1066.

GILL, O. N., SOCKETT, P. N., BARTLETT, C. L. R., VAILE, M. S. B., ROWE, B., GILBERT, R. J., DULAKE, C., MURRELL, H. C. & SALMASO, S. 1983 Outbreak of *Salmonella napoli* infection caused by contaminated chocolate bars. *Lancet* **i**, 574–577.

HALL, L. P. 1982 *A Manual of Methods for the Bacteriological Examination of Frozen Foods*. Oxford: Oxford University Press.

INTERNATIONAL STANDARDS ORGANISATION. 1981 Methods for microbiological examination of food and animal feeding stuffs. Part 4. Detection of *Salmonella*. *British Standard 5763: 1982*. ISO 6579–1981.

KRYSINSKI, E. P. & HEIMSCH, R. C. 1977 Use of enzyme-labelled antibodies to detect *Salmonella* in foods. *Applied and Environmental Microbiology* **33**, 947–954.

MATTINGLY, J. A. 1984 An enzyme immunoassay for the detection of all *Salmonella* using a combination of a myeloma protein and a hybridoma antibody. *Journal of Immunological Methods* **73**, 147–156.

MATTINGLY, J. A. & GEHLE, W. D. 1984 An improved immunoassay for the detection of *Salmonella*. *Journal of Food Science* **49**, 807–809.

MATTINGLY, J. A., ROBISON, B. J., BOEHM, A. & GEHLE, W. D. 1985 Use of monoclonal antibodies for the detection of *Salmonella* in foods. *Journal of Food Technology* **39**, 90–94.

MINNICH, S. A. 1978 *The Detection of Salmonella in Foods by Using Enzyme-Labelled Antibodies*. M.Sc. Thesis University of Idaho.

MINNICH, S. A., HARTMAN, P. A. & HEIMSCH, R. C. 1982 Enzyme immunoassay for detection of salmonellae in foods. *Applied and Environmental Microbiology* **43**, 877–883.

MMWR 1986 Foodborne disease outbreaks, Annual Summary, 1982. *Centers for Disease Control, Surveillance Summaries 1986* **35**(155), 755–1655.

ROBISON, B. J., PRETZMAN, C. I. & MATTINGLY, J. A. 1983 Enzyme immunoassay in which a myeloma protein is used for detection of *Salmonellae*. *Applied and Environmental Microbiology* **45**, 1816–1821.

SWAMINATHAN, B. & AYRES, J. C. 1980 A direct immunoenzyme method for the detection of salmonellae in foods. *Journal of Food Science* **45**, 352–361.

TODD, L. S., ROBERTS, D., BARTHOLOMEW, B. A. & GILBERT, R. J. 1986 Evaluation of an enzyme immunoassay kit for the detection of salmonellae in foods and feeds. *Proceedings of the Second World Congress on Foodborne Infections and Intoxications, 1986*. **Volume 1**: 418–421. Berlin Institute of Veterinary Medicine/Robert von Ostertag-Institute.

WORLD HEALTH ORGANIZATION 1982 *WHO Surveillance Programme for Control of Foodborne Infections and Intoxications in Europe*. Third report. Geneva: WHO.

ELISA Techniques for the Detection of Sulphate-Reducing Bacteria

CHRISTINE GAYLARDE AND PAUL COOK

City of London Polytechnic, Department of Biological Sciences, Old Castle Street, London E1 7NT

Introduction

The sulphate-reducing bacteria

The sulphate-reducing bacteria (SRB) are a group of anaerobic, heterotrophic organisms, abundant in the natural environment, which are responsible for a number of economic problems. Their peculiar metabolism leads to the production of vast amounts of hydrogen sulphide gas. This can cause spoilage of canned foods, in which the genus *Desulfotomaculum* has been implicated, or the corrosion of metal structures in anaerobic areas such as some soils and aqueous sediments.

The genus *Desulfovibrio* and the more recently discovered SRB such as *Desulfobacter* and *Desulfobulbus* are of great importance in the offshore oil industry (Hamilton, 1983), where they may cause the souring of crude oil and health hazards on the platforms, quite apart from their corrosive activities. The production of ferrous sulphides in anaerobic areas by SRB, may also induce blockages of oil-bearing strata, filters and valves, etc. The industries in which SRB cause significant problems are very diverse. Some of these are indicated in Table 1.

The label 'sulphate-reducing bacteria' is reserved for a group of organisms which carry out dissimilatory sulphate reduction. Inorganic sulphur, in one of its oxidized states, is utilized by the cells as a terminal electron acceptor, consequently becoming reduced to sulphide. The most common form of sulphur utilized by the cells is sulphate and the first step in its reduction is the formation of adenosine phosphosulphate, with the utilization of energy, in the form of ATP. Together with subsequent electron transfers, leading to the final production of sulphide, this results in rather limited energy being made available to the cells when compared with an aerobic type of metabolism. In addition, the SRB have limited nutritional sources, being able to use only a small range of carbon-containing compounds (Postgate, 1984). Thus the cultivation of this group of bacteria in the laboratory is far from trouble-free. The various media available for their growth, all somewhat complex,

TABLE 1.　*Incidence of SRB-related problems*

Industry	Nature of problems
Major problems	
Offshore oil	Corrosion of pipes and storage tanks. Blockage of filters and valves. Souring of oil. Health risks
Onshore oil	Corrosion of tanks and valves. Contamination of stored oil and fuels
Gas	Corrosion of metal tanks and pipes. Contamination of gas
Water	Corrision of pipes, valves, heat exchangers and storage tanks. Objectionable odours
Metal working	Corrosion of tools and products. Blackening of emulsions, paintwork and metal. Objectionable odours
Minor problems	
Paper	Blackening of pulp
Food	Spoilage of canned vegetables and molasses
Leather	Blackening of leather during tanning
Adhesives & paints	Blackening of product

have recently been reviewed by Herbert & Gilbert (1984). These authors point out that the two commercially available media have only limited usefulness.

The adverse effects of the presence of SRB in a number of situations means that it is important not only to be able to detect their presence and activity but also to be able to assess the efficacy of any eradication treatment. The achievement of both of these is made more difficult by the capricious nature of the organisms, in addition to the necessity for choosing appropriate media and conditions of incubation for growth. Thus, reliable methods for the detection and enumeration of SRB are few and mostly require prolonged incubation periods in specialized media and the maintenance of anaerobic conditions. One of the most frequently used methods is the most probable number technique (MPN), which involves the preparation of large quantities of appropriate media and the maintenance of anaerobic conditions throughout the whole procedure. Incubation periods are, at a minimum, 3 days and results should not be recorded as negative until 4 weeks after inoculation.

The use of ELISA techniques for SRB assay offers the possibility of rapid and extremely sensitive enumeration methods, which do not involve the culture of the organisms and hence avoid the need for choice of suitable medium and long incubation periods. In addition, no facilities for anaerobic incubation are required.

ELISA techniques

The development of the quantitative ELISA method stems from the work of Engvall & Perlmann (1971) and Van Weemen & Schuurs (1971), who developed the early solid phase enzyme immunoassays. Since then microtitre plates have become increasingly popular as the solid phase. Two types of assay are commonly used: the direct and indirect types. The direct, or double antibody sandwich (DAS), form involves coating the wells of a microtitre plate with specific antibody, incubating with the sample under test and then detecting any specifically-bound antigen with enzyme-conjugated specific antibody which itself is detected by the addition of an enzyme-specific substrate which reacts with the enzyme to form a coloured product. This technique has been widely used for detecting a variety of antigens, including plant viruses (Clark & Adams, 1977), *Rhizobium* spp. (Kishinevsky & Bar-Joseph, 1978) and the fungus *Epichloë typhina* (Johnson *et al.*, 1982). The indirect ELISA technique uses the alternative strategy of coating the test sample containing antigen onto the wells of the microtitre plate. Specific antibody (IgG) is then added and this is detected by the addition of enzyme-labelled anti-IgG followed by the enzyme substrate. Micro-organisms which have been detected by an indirect ELISA method include *Salmonella* (Krysinski & Heimsch, 1977) and tobacco mosaic virus (Van Regenmortel & Burckard, 1980).

The most significant characteristic of immunosorbant assays is their high sensitivity, enabling the detection of lower concentrations of antigens than most other methods (Clark, 1981). Additionally, they have the ability to be extremely specific. It has been stated that the direct ELISA technique is more efficient in this respect, showing a very narrow strain specificity in virus assays (Van Regenmortel & Burckard, 1980).

Both ELISA and radioimmunoassay (RIA) techniques are suitable immunological methods for highly sensitive assays. However, the ELISA is probably more appropriate for most uses and certainly for field tests outside the laboratory, as it achieves the high sensitivity associated with RIA without the expense and safety hazards of radioisotope work.

The ELISA techniques described in this communication include the immobilization onto plates of both antisera and antigens. The method chosen will depend upon the level of specificity and speed of result required.

Materials and Methods

Growth and preparation of SRB antigens for immunization of rabbits

SRB are grown in Postgate's medium C (Postgate, 1984) in batch culture at 30 °C. After 5 days, the cells are harvested by centrifugation at 3000 rpm for 30 min at 4 °C. After washing twice in phosphate-buffered saline (PBS) containing 0.14 M sodium chloride and 25 mM phosphate buffer pH 7.4, the final pellet of cells is resuspended in PBS and a sample is removed for enumeration using a haemocytometer. The concentration is then adjusted to around 10^9 cells/ml using PBS.

Immunization procedure

Sixteen strains of SRB have been used to raise antisera in New Zealand white rabbits. The exact number and types of SRB used will depend upon the purpose for which the assay is to be used. Rabbits are bled to obtain pre-immune serum and then injected with 1 ml of the SRB cell suspension, prepared as above, mixed with 1 ml of Freund's Complete Adjuvant. Inoculation is repeated at 10 and 20 days, when the incomplete adjuvant replaces the complete form. Blood samples are obtained from the marginal ear vein of the rabbits after 27 days and thereafter at weekly intervals. They are left to clot overnight at 4 °C and the serum is then collected and stored at −20 °C.

Determination of antibody titre and preparation of polyvalent antiserum

Titres of the antisera are measured by whole cell agglutinations in microtitre plates. Sera are diluted twofold in 22 wells of the plate using PBS as diluent. An equal volume of antigen (10^9 cells/ml in PBS) is added and the plates are incubated at 4 °C overnight. The antibody titre is given as the reciprocal of the last dilution showing agglutination. Sera may be used individually if enumeration of a known species is required, or mixed to produce a polyvalent antiserum which will detect a range of strains, species, or genera. The polyvalent antiserum is produced by adjusting the agglutination titre of each individual serum to 4096 and mixing in equal volumes. Alternatively, a polyvalent antiserum may be produced by using the ELISA technique to determine antibody titre prior to mixing.

The ELISA techniques

The direct ELISA

1 Microtitre plates are incubated with antibody (salt-precipitated dialysed protein from the antiserum, concentration adjusted to 5 μg/ml) in 50 mM carbonate buffer pH 9.6 for 3 h at 37 °C.

2 Plates are washed three times, for 3 min each time, with PBS–Tween 20 0.05% to remove excess antibody.

3 The sample under test is added, diluted where necessary in PBS–Tween 20, 0.1%; polyvinylpyrrolidone (PVP), 2% and bovine serum albumin (BSA), 2%. Incubation is at 37 °C overnight or 37 °C for 3 h followed by 4 °C overnight.

4 After washing the plates three times for 3 min each time in PBS–Tween 20, 0.1%; BSA, 0.5%; PVP, 0.5% and EDTA, 2 mM, specific antibody which has been conjugated to the enzyme peroxidase is added. This is prepared by the periodate method (Wilson & Nakane, 1978) and diluted to 1:250 in the washing solution detailed in step 4 with EDTA omitted. Incubation is for 3–4 h at 37 °C.

5 Plates are washed three times in PBS–Tween 20, 0.1% and the enzyme substrate is then added. This is prepared as follows: 1.009 g 3,3′–5,5′ tetramethylbenzidine

(TMP) is dissolved in 100 ml dimethyl sulphoxide and 10 ml of this is added to 1 litre of sodium acetate—citric acid buffer pH 5.5. Hydrogen peroxide is added to a final concentration of 1.3 mM. Incubation is for 1 h at room temperature.

6 The reaction is stopped with 12.5% sulphuric acid and the absorbance read at 450 nm.

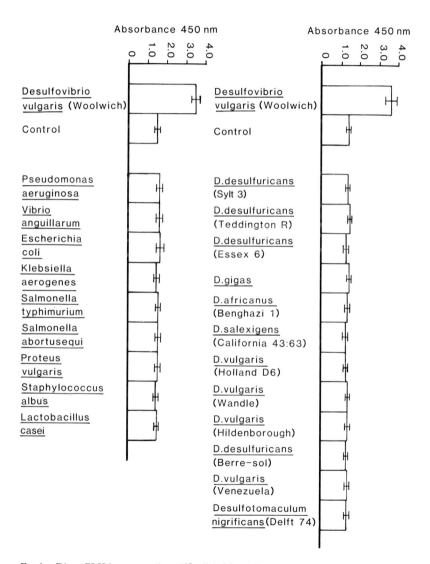

FIG. 1.   Direct ELISA cross reactions. 10⁷ cells/ml for each type.

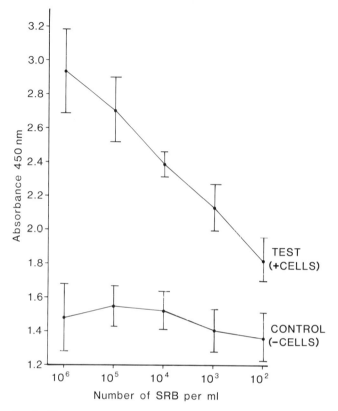

FIG. 2.   Direct ELISA standard curve for *D. vulgaris* (Woolwich).

    This technique is recommended for the detection and enumeration of single species or strains of SRB. Figure 1 shows that there is very little cross-reaction between strains of SRB or with other genera when a monovalent antiserum is used. The method is easily able to detect 10^3 cells/ml (Fig. 2) and could probably be used for more dilute samples.

    Polyvinylpyrrolidone (PVP) is reported to decrease non-specific background reactions (Hill, 1984). In spite of its use in this method, rather high control readings are obtained. This may be due to the presence of residual unconjugated peroxidase and the assay may be improved by purification of the conjugate prior to use.

    Several authors have reported a high degree of strain specificity in direct ELISA techniques (van Regenmortel & Burckard, 1980; Nambiar & Anjaiah, 1985). The present method, although unsuitable for the detection of a range of SRB, does have the advantage of a high degree of specificity. Such a strain-specific test could be used alongside activity measurements, for example, the radiorespirometric assay of sulphate reduction (Hardy & Syrett, 1983), for examining biocide sensitivity.

Battersby *et al.* (1985) have described the possible resistance of SRB to a number of cationic biocides and there may be an increasing need in the future to be able to monitor the effects of biocides administered over any length of time.

The indirect ELISA

In the indirect ELISA technique, the specific anti-bacterial serum is unlabelled and is detected by the addition of a second anti-species IgG antibody which is enzyme-conjugated. This modification is claimed to give higher sensitivity and reduced specificity (Bar-Joseph & Malkinson, 1980). The technique used for SRB is detailed below.

1 Samples concentrated by centrifugation or diluted if necessary in carbonate buffer are applied to the wells of a microtitre plate and incubated at 37 °C overnight or at 37 °C for 3 h and 4 °C overnight.
2 After incubation, plates are washed in phosphate buffered saline, pH 7.4, containing Tween 20, 0.05%, for 3 min. This washing procedure is repeated three times.
3 Plates are incubated for 1 h at 37 °C with 1% bovine serum albumin (BSA) to block non-specific binding sites and then washed in PBS-Tween 20 as previously.
4 Antiserum (either monovalent or polyvalent) diluted in PBS-Tween 20, 0.1% is added to the wells and incubated at 37 °C for 3–4 h followed by 4 °C overnight.
5 Plates are washed three times for 3 min each in PBS-Tween 20, 0.1%; BSA, 0.5%; PVP, 0.5% and EDTA 2 mM.
6 Goat anti-rabbit IgG conjugated to horseradish peroxidase (Sigma) is diluted 1:1000 in the washing mixture used in step 5 without the EDTA component. This is added to the wells and incubated at 37 °C for 3 h.
7 Plates are washed as before in PBS-Tween 20, 0.1%, and the succeeding steps applied as in the previous method.

This technique provides an extremely sensitive method, allowing the detection of 10^2 cells/ml (Fig. 3). The time taken to perform the assay (results obtainable in 45–48 h) offers a considerable saving over the MPN method which may require 4 weeks for a result if SRB numbers are low. Ideally the polyvalent antiserum used for the ELISA should detect all strains of SRB. The present studies have been limited to an antiserum containing antibodies directed against seven types of *Desulfovibrio*, but it is proposed to extend this to 16 or 17 types of SRB so that most industrially important strains will be detected.

The use of polyvalent antisera containing antibodies to a single genus or even a single species of SRB, combined with the radiorespirometric method for the determination of sulphate-reducing activity (Rosser & Hamilton, 1983), using a variety of carbon substrates (lactate, pyruvate, formate and acetate), would enable the genus or species of SRB active in particular environments to be ascertained. Such studies could be completed much more rapidly with these techniques than has

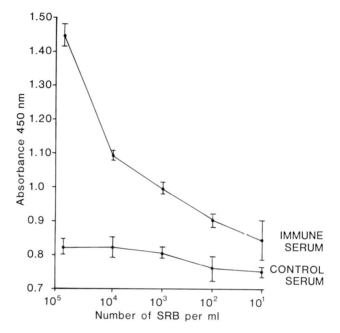

FIG. 3.   Indirect ELISA standard curve for *D. vulgaris* (Woolwich).

previously been possible. It is known that certain species of SRB are more resistant to inhibition than others (Al-Hitti *et al.*, 1983). The potential to identify rapidly SRB types causing problems in a particular area would mean that individual programmes of treatment could be designed, much like the situation in clinical microbiology.

The modified indirect ELISA

Although the previous method is extremely sensitive, a relatively lengthy incubation period is required to ensure efficient immobilization of the bacteria in the sample to the microtitre plate support. This immobilization period can be shortened by the use of titanous hydroxide, which has previously been shown to be an efficient solid phase for immobilization of bacterial cells in polystyrene tubes (Ibrahim *et al.*, 1985). The microtitre plates used routinely in the City of London Polytechnic laboratory are flat-bottomed Nunc-Immuno II plates and for SRB the optimum volume of titanous hydroxide has been determined to be around one fifth of the sample volume (Fig. 4). Round-bottomed wells (LIP plates) can also be used and it

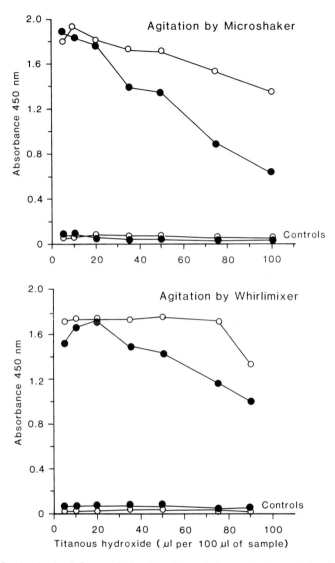

FIG. 4. Graphs showing influence of microtitre plate well shape, agitation method and quantity of titanous hydroxide on efficiency of immobilization of SRB (Woolwich strain, 10^8 cells/ml) as detected by the modified indirect ELISA. Test wells received polyvalent antiserum (Strains 1–3 and 5–8, Fig. 6) and control wells pre-immune serum. Each point is the mean of four replicates. ●–●–● microtitre plate with flat-bottomed wells. ○–○–○ microtitre plate with round-bottomed wells.

may be that in these immobilization is more efficient (Fig. 4). The method for SRB detection* is as follows:

1 Microtitre plates are incubated with samples concentrated or diluted as required in 0.85% sodium chloride.

2 For each 100 μl of sample, 20 μl titanous hydroxide suspension prepared as described by Ibrahim *et al.* (1985), is added and the plates are shaken for 30 min at room temperature.

3 Plates are washed three times, each time for a period of 3 min, in casein buffer (10 mM Tris hydrochloric acid pH 7.6 containing 154 mM sodium chloride and 0.5% casein).

4 Antiserum is diluted 1:250 in casein buffer and applied to the wells of the plates, which are then incubated at 55 °C for 90 min.

5 After washing three times for 3 min each time in casein buffer, goat anti-rabbit IgG conjugated to horseradish peroxidase (Sigma Chemical Co. Ltd., Poole, Dorset), diluted 1:500 in casein buffer, is added to each well and the plates incubated at 37 °C for 2.5 h.

6 Plates are washed as before in PBS containing 0.14 M sodium chloride and 25 mM phosphate buffer pH 7.4 and the enzyme substrate is then added as in the previous methods.

Although somewhat less sensitive than the unmodified indirect ELISA (Fig. 5), this method provides a much more rapid result, with the assay being completed

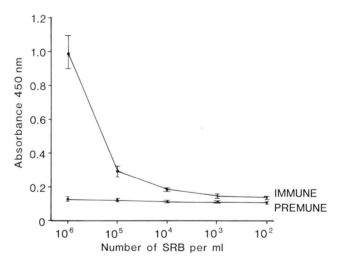

FIG. 5. Modified indirect ELISA standard curve for *D. vulgaris* (Woolwich). Polyvalent antiserum containing antibodies raised agsinst seven strains.

* Patent application filed.

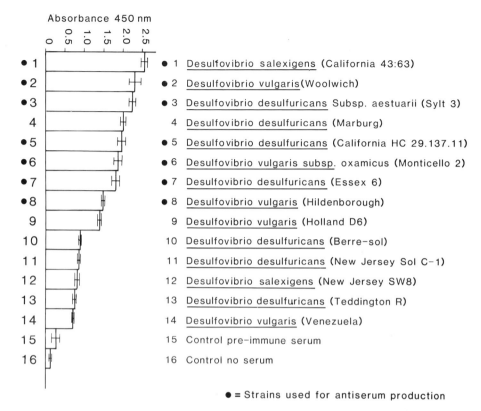

Absorbance 450 nm

● = Strains used for antiserum production

FIG. 6.   Modified indirect ELISA cross-reactions with related SRB. 10⁷ cells/ml for each type.

within a working day. The cross-reactions with other SRB (Fig. 6) are sufficiently strong to allow its use, with the sevenfold polyvalent antiserum, for general SRB detection. The addition of antibodies raised against other SRB, especially numbers 10 to 14 in Fig. 6, should enable many of the environmentally important strains to be enumerated. The cross-reactions with non-SRB are minimal (Fig. 7), indicating a degree of specificity ideal for testing environmental samples.

Discussion and Conclusions

The ELISA techniques are seen to be very sensitive and to give results within 2 days rather than the weeks required for traditional culture tests. The small degree of cross-reaction seen in the direct, or double antibody sandwich technique suggests that this method would be suitable for the detection and enumeration of specific

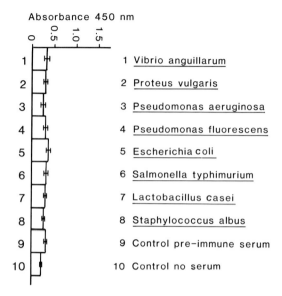

Absorbance 450 nm

1 Vibrio anguillarum
2 Proteus vulgaris
3 Pseudomonas aeruginosa
4 Pseudomonas fluorescens
5 Escherichia coli
6 Salmonella typhimurium
7 Lactobacillus casei
8 Staphylococcus albus
9 Control pre-immune serum
10 Control no serum

FIG. 7.   Modified indirect ELISA cross reactions with non-SRB genera. 10^7 cells for each type.

TABLE 2.   *Comparative counts of SRB obtained using the MPN and modified indirect ELISA methods*

| | Number of SRB/ml as determined by | |
Sample no.	MPN technique*	ELISA method†
1	4	182
2	8	132
3	133	3155
4	2	1656
5	2	6011
6	4	9418
7	0	2 8117
8	0	8298
9	0	1377

Samples used were water from an oil production platform using secondary recovery. They were concentrated ten times by centrifugation prior to use in the test.

* All handling and manipulation of samples were performed in an anaerobic cabinet. Growth medium was Postgate's medium B (Postgate, 1984) made up in 3 parts North Sea water to 1 part distilled water pH 7.3. Incubation time was 28 days.

† Polyvalent antiserum against strains 1–3 and 5–8 (Fig. 6) was used.

strains of SRB, whilst the indirect techniques are applicable to total SRB enumeration.

The modified ELISA, whilst not at present having the sensitivity of the unmodified form, is much more rapid, results being available within 6 h. The use of titanous hydroxide causes a rapid immobilization of bacterial cells, thus reducing the duration of the first step in the procedure. It seems unlikely that the detection of low numbers of cells will be essential for routine testing, although the concentration of cells which can initiate problems has not been defined. However, the modified test could doubtless be made more sensitive if required.

It has been shown that ELISA techniques may be used to enumerate specific bacterial genera within mixed populations (Archer, 1984). Our tests confirm that this is possible for SRB. Table 2 gives a comparison of SRB counts obtained from various North Sea platform water samples using the modified ELISA and the MPN technique. It is obvious that many more cells are detected by the ELISA. No relationship is seen between the counts obtained by the two methods. This reflects, in part at least, the unreliable nature of the MPN test. Many of the organisms detected by ELISA may have been unable to grow in the medium used for the MPN.

The use of ELISA techniques for SRB detection allows significant improvements over conventional methods in speed of results, sensitivity and handling time for multiple specimens and its use will certainly increase in the future.

References

AL-HITTI, I. K., MOODY, G. J. & THOMAS, J. D. R. 1983 Sulphide ion-selective electrode studies concerning *Desulfovibrio* species of sulphate-reducing bacteria. *Analyst* **108**, 1209–1220.

ARCHER, D. B. 1984 Detection and quantitation of methanogens by ELISA. *Applied and Environmental Microbiology* **48**, 797–801.

BAR-JOSEPH, M. & MALKINSON, M. 1980 Hen egg yolk as a source of antiviral antibodies in the ELISA: a comparison of two plant viruses. *Journal of Virological Methods* **1**, 179–183.

BATTERSBY, N. S., STEWART, D. J. & SHARMA, A. P. 1985 Microbiological problems in the offshore oil and gas industries. *Journal of Applied Bacteriology Symposium Supplement 1985*, 227S–253S.

CLARK, M. F. 1981 Immunosorbant assays in plant pathology. *Annual Review of Phytopathology* **19**, 83–106.

CLARK, M. F. & ADAMS, A. N. 1977 Characteristics of the microplate method of ELISA for the detection of plant viruses. *Journal of general Virology* **34**, 475–483.

ENGVALL, E. & PERLMANN, F. 1971 ELISA quantitative assay of IgG. *Immunochemistry* **8**, 871–874.

HAMILTON, W. A. 1983 The sulphate-reducing bacteria: their physiology and subsequent ecology. In *Microbial Corrosion*, pp. 1–5. London: The Metals Society.

HARDY, J. A. & SYRETT, K. R. 1983 A radiorespirometric method for evaluating inhibitors of sulphate-reducing bacteria. *European Journal of Applied Microbiology and Biotechnology* **17**, 49–52.

HERBERT, B. N. & GILBERT, P. D. 1984 Isolation and growth of sulphate-reducing bacteria. In *Microbiological Methods for Environmental Biotechnology* eds. Granger, J. M. & Lynch, J. M. pp. 235–257. London: Academic Press.

HILL, S. 1984 The ELISA technique for the detection of plant viruses. In *Microbiological Methods for Environmental Biotechnology* eds. Grainger, J. M. & LYNCH, J. M. pp. 349–363. London: Academic Press.

IBRAHIM, G. F., LYONS, M. J., WALKER, R. A. & FLEET, G. H. 1985 Immobilisation of microorganisms for detection by solid-phase immunoassays. *Journal of Clinical Microbiology* 22, 361–365.

JOHNSON, M. C., PIRONE, T. P., SIEGEL, M. R. & VARNEY, D. R. 1982 Detection of *Epichloë typhina* in tall fesule by means of ELISA. *Phytopathology* 72, 647–649.

KISHINEVSKY, B. & BAR-JOSEPH, M. 1978 *Rhizobium* strain identification in *Arachis hypogaea* nodules by ELISA. *Canadian Journal of Microbiology* 24, 1537–1543.

KRYSINSKI, E. P. & HEIMSCH, R. C. 1977 Use of enzyme-labelled antibodies to detect *Salmonella* in foods. *Applied and Environmental Microbiology* 33, 947–954.

NAMBIAR, P. T. C. & ANJAIAH, V. 1985 Enumeration of rhizobia by ELISA. *Journal of Applied Bacteriology* 58, 187–193.

POSTGATE, J. R. 1984 *The Sulphate-reducing Bacteria.* Cambridge: Cambridge University Press.

ROSSER, H. R. & HAMILTON, W. A. 1983 Simplified assay for accurate determination of ^{35}S-sulphate reduction activity. *Applied and Environmental Microbiology* 45, 1956–1959.

VAN REGENMORTEL, M. H. V. & BURCKARD, J. 1980 Detection of a wide spectrum of tobacco mosaic virus strains by indirect ELISAs. *Virology* 106, 327–334.

VAN WEEMEN, B. K. & SCHUURS, A. H. W. M. 1971 Immunoassay using antigen-enzyme conjugates. *FEBS Letters* 15, 232–236.

WILSON, M. B. & NAKANE, P. K. 1978 Recent developments in the periodate method of conjugating horseradish peroxidase (HRPO) to antibodies. In *Immunofluorescence and Related Staining Techniques* eds. Knapp, W., Holubar, K. & Wicks, G. Amsterdam: Elsevier.

Use of Commercial Kits for the Detection of *Clostridium perfringens* and *Staphylococcus aureus* Enterotoxins

P. R. BERRY, ANTONNETTE A. WIENEKE, JOANNA C. RODHOUSE AND
R. J. GILBERT

*Food Hygiene Laboratory, Central Public Health Laboratory, 61 Colindale Ave, London
NW9 5HT*

Introduction

Clostridium perfringens

Food poisoning due to *C. perfringens* occurs after the ingestion of food containing large numbers of vegetative cells (Hobbs *et al.*, 1953; Sutton & Hobbs, 1968). The organism multiplies and sporulates in the intestine, and when the mature spores are released from the sporangia there is an accompanying release of enterotoxin. It is this toxin that is responsible for the typical symptoms of *C. perfringens* food poisoning.

An outbreak due to *C. perfringens* is confirmed in the laboratory when at least one of the following criteria are satisfied (Stringer *et al.*, 1982): (1) the incriminated food, correctly stored after the incident, contains $\geqslant 10^5$ *C. perfringens*/g; (2) the median faecal spore count is $\geqslant 10^6$/g; (3) strains isolated from the incriminated food and faecal specimens belong to the same serotype; and (4) isolates from the faeces of most of the patients belong to the same serotype.

Although extremely valuable, these criteria may on occasion be unhelpful: (1) when the incriminated food has been stored frozen or for long periods (i.e. over 48 h) resulting in a decrease in viable vegetative cells; (2) when faecal specimens have been collected several days after onset of symptoms resulting in a decrease in the faecal spore count, and re-establishment of the patients' own serotypes; (3) when the isolated strains are non-typable; and (4) when dealing with geriatric long-stay hospital patients, who may carry large numbers of the same serotype in the absence of diarrhoea (Stringer *et al.*, 1985).

It is because of these problems, together with the time required for isolation, purification and serotyping, that demonstration of the enterotoxin in faeces has become a valuable adjunct in the confirmation of *C. perfringens* food poisoning outbreaks.

Several methods (reviewed by Stringer, 1985) have been developed for the

Immunological Techniques
in Microbiology
0–632–01908–5

245

detection of *C. perfringens* enterotoxin. An immunological assay using ELISA is probably the method of choice, being sensitive, specific, reproducible and rapid, as well as providing a quantitative result (Bartholomew *et al.*, 1985; Wimsatt *et al.*, 1986). There are, however, two disadvantages—the test requires specialized equipment (e.g. microplate reader) for optimum sensitivity, and also some expertise particularly if reagents are prepared 'in-house'.

Recently, workers in Japan developed a reversed passive latex agglutination (RPLA) test for the detection of *C. perfringens* enterotoxin. The test is now available in kit form, has a reported sensitivity of 2 ng of toxin/g of faeces, and requires no specialized equipment.

Since the method appeared to offer a useful semi-quantitative alternative to our standard microplate ELISA, the kit was evaluated over a period of 12 months on faecal specimens submitted from cases of suspected *C. perfringens* food poisoning.

Staphylococcus aureus

Staphylococcal food poisoning is an acute gastroenteritis following the ingestion of a food containing enterotoxin(s) produced by a strain of *Staphylococcus aureus* in that food. So far five different enterotoxins have been identified: enterotoxin A (SEA), B (SEB), C (SEC), D (SED) and E (SEE).

An outbreak of food poisoning is considered to be caused by staphylococcal enterotoxin when, in addition to typical symptoms and incubation times, large numbers of an enterotoxigenic strain of *S. aureus* ($> 10^6$/g) are found in the implicated food and/or a similar strain is isolated from faecal and vomitus specimens. Better proof of an outbreak, however, is the detection of enterotoxin in the food itself. In the past a gel diffusion test was used for the detection of enterotoxin in the foods (Gilbert *et al.*, 1972). Because of the small amounts of enterotoxin present, a lengthy extraction and concentration procedure was needed to prepare a food for testing. Recently ELISA and RPLA tests have been developed which are more sensitive than the gel diffusion method and require simpler extraction procedures.

The ELISA developed by Fey *et al.* (1984) and the RPLA test developed by Shingaki *et al.* (1981) (Igarashi *et al.*, 1985), are now commercially available in kit form. In this study the efficiency of the two kits in detecting staphylococcal enterotoxins in foods from outbreaks of food poisoning in the U.K. was determined. The results were compared to those obtained with the plate-ELISA (Notermans *et al.*, 1983; Wieneke & Gilbert, 1985).

Materials and Methods

Clostridium perfringens enterotoxin

Faecal specimens

For evaluation of the *C. perfringens* RPLA kit, test materials were faecal specimens from suspected outbreaks of *C. perfringens* food poisoning. The specimens were sent to the Food Hygiene Laboratory for enterotoxin tests by Public Health Laboratory Service and hospital laboratories in the U.K. between August 1985 and July 1986.

Extraction of enterotoxin

Faeces, 3–4 g, were homogenized in 3–4 ml 0.01 M phosphate buffer pH 7.2 containing 0.15 M sodium chloride (PBS). The suspension was centrifuged at 13 000 g for 20 min at 4 °C, and the supernatant fluid was filtered through a 0.2 μm membrane filter. The filtrate was used as the test material.

Detection of enterotoxin

1 *ELISA*: the assay procedure was carried out as described by Bartholomew *et al.* (1985).
2 *Reversed passive latex agglutination* (RPLA): the RPLA kits were purchased from Denka-Seiken Co. Ltd., Tokyo, Japan, but are now available from Oxoid Ltd., Basingstoke, England (Code no. DR930).

The test was carried out in round-bottomed microtitre plates (Microtitre, Dynatech Lab. Ltd., Billingshurst, Sussex), using the kit and its instructions. The kit consists of one bottle each of suspensions of sensitized (anti-enterotoxin) and control (normal rabbit immunoglobulin) latex, diluent, and freeze dried enterotoxin as control. Each sample required two rows of wells. A twofold dilution series of the faecal extract was made across each row. An aliquot (25 μl) of sensitized latex was added to each well of the first row, and 25 μl of control latex added to each well of the second row. Positive and negative controls were set up using purified enterotoxin with the control and sensitized latex. The plate was shaken on a plate shaker for about 10 s, then covered and incubated at room temperature overnight.

Agglutination reactions were scored as + + + (complete agglutination), + +, +, ±, or −, with ± and − being judged negative. A specimen was considered to contain *C. perfringens* enterotoxin when the positive agglutination in the sensitized row exceeded that in the control row by two or more wells.

Neutralization of latex agglutination

Faecal extract was added to an equal volume of either normal rabbit serum or rabbit anti-enterotoxin diluted 1:5 in diluent. The mixture was incubated at room temperature for 30 min and then tested as described.

Staphylococcal enterotoxins

Foods

The staphylococcal enterotoxin detection kits were tested on foods from 27 suspected outbreaks of staphylococcal food poisoning. The foods were sent to the

Food Hygiene Laboratory, Colindale, for enterotoxin tests by Public Health Laboratory Service and hospital laboratories in the U.K. from June 1981 to September 1986. A further 20 foods unconnected with staphylococcal food poisoning were also examined.

ENUMERATION OF *S. AUREUS* IN FOODS

The number of *S. aureus* present in the foods was determined on Baird-Parker agar (CM 275 Oxoid Ltd, England) using a surface drop method. Colonies were confirmed as *S. aureus* by coagulase production in 10% plasma broth.

Extraction of enterotoxins

Samples of food (10–100 g) were homogenized with equal amounts of distilled water and the pH of the food slurry was adjusted to 4.5 with 2 M hydrochloric acid (Reiser *et al.*, 1974; Wieneke & Gilbert, 1985). Some of the food slurries were centrifuged at 15 000 g for 20 min before acidification of the supernatent fluids to pH 4.5. The acidified food slurry or extract was centrifuged at 15 000 g for 20 min, the supernatant fluid taken off and the pH adjusted to 7.5 with 5 M sodium hydroxide. If a precipitate formed, the extract was centrifuged again. The extract was shaken with 20% of its volume of chloroform and after centrifugation at 2500 g for 10 min the upper (aqueous) layer was used with the ELISA and RPLA kits. In the plate ELISA the extract was tested both unconcentrated and concentrated 5 to 10 times.

Detection of enterotoxins

1 *Gel diffusion:* the gel-diffusion method (Gilbert *et al.*, 1972) was used for the detection of enterotoxin (SEA to SEE) production by strains of *S. aureus* isolated from the foods under investigation.

2 *Plate ELISA:* the plate ELISA was carried out as described by Notermans *et al.* (1983) and Wieneke & Gilbert (1985). Antibodies to staphylococcal enterotoxin were raised in sheep and microtitre plates were used as the solid phase. Foods were examined for the presence of SEA or SEB or both depending on the enterotoxin produced by the *S. aureus* strain isolated from the food. In two cases where *S. aureus* was not detected in the food from an outbreak, the extracts were only tested for SEA.

3 *ELISA kit:* the ELISA kit was obtained from Labor Dr W. Bommeli, Länggass strasse 7, CH-3012 Bern, Switzerland.

One ELISA kit contains reagents sufficient for 10 tests for each of four enterotoxins (SEA to SED). It includes colour-coded polystyrene beads coated with anti-SEA, -SEB, -SEC and -SED IgG (10 of each), 20 control beads coated with normal rabbit serum (NRS) IgG, anti-SE-alkaline phosphatase conjugates (8 ml of each anti-SE), NRS, 10 × concentrated wash solution, substrate (p-nitrophenyl phosphate) tablets and buffer.

The kit instructions were followed with a few minor modifications (Wieneke & Gilbert, 1987). Twenty millilitres of the prepared 1:2 food extracts were incubated with NRS (final concentration 2.5%) and Tween 20 (final concentration 0.25%) at room temperature for 30 min and centrifuged at 25 000 g for 20 min. Antibody coated beads (one of each kind) and four control beads were added to the supernatant fluid in a flask prerinsed with wash solution. After incubation with gentle shaking at room temperature overnight the beads were washed four times with the wash solution: each bead was transferred to a separate 4 ml polystyrene tube prewashed with the wash solution and 0.45 ml of each of the four conjugates was added to the corresponding antibody-coated bead and to one control bead. After incubation at room temperature for 6 h the beads were washed as before and 0.9 ml of substrate dissolved in buffer was added to each bead. After 1 h at room temperature, 0.2 ml quantities were removed from the tubes, placed in the wells of a microtitre plate and the absorbance at 405 nm was determined with a microtitre plate reader. If many samples are tested the enzyme reaction can be stopped by adding 0.1 ml of 2 M sodium hydroxide to the reaction mixture.

Foods which contained enterotoxigenic strains of *S. aureus* were only tested for the presence of the enterotoxin(s) produced by the strain. Other foods were tested for the presence of all four enterotoxins.

4 *Reversed passive latex agglutination:* the RPLA kit was obtained from Denka-Seiken Co. Ltd, Japan, but is now available from Oxoid Ltd, England (Code no. DR 900).

One RPLA kit contains reagents sufficient for 20 tests for each of four enterotoxins (SEA to SED). It includes four antibody-coated latex suspensions (one for each enterotoxin), an NRS IgG-coated latex suspension, freeze-dried reference enterotoxins and dilution buffer.

In this study the 1:2 food extracts prepared for the ELISA were used in the RPLA test. The manufacturer recommends a 1:10 food extract in saline. Five identical rows of doubling dilutions of the extract in the buffer provided were prepared over 4–6 wells in a 96 well round-bottomed microtitre plate (0.02 ml final volumes). To the wells in each of the rows one drop of one of the sensitized latex suspensions, or of the control latex suspension, was added. The plate was shaken well and incubated at room temperature overnight. The purified enterotoxins were used as positive controls. The agglutination reactions were scored as for the *C. perfringens* RPLA kit. Positive results were confirmed by neutralization of the enterotoxin in the extract with 0.1% of the corresponding antiserum.

All foods were tested for the presence of SEA, SEB and SEC. Reagents for the detection of SED became available in October 1985. Many food extracts were no longer available by that time and therefore only some of the food extracts were tested for the presence of SED.

Results and Discussion

Clostridium perfringens

Two hundred and seventy four faecal specimens from 55 separate outbreaks of suspected *C. perfringens* food poisoning were examined by both ELISA and RPLA. The results are summarized in Table 1 and show that 254 (93%) of specimens gave the same results in both tests. The discrepancy that arose in 20 of the specimens was considered to be due to very low toxin levels ($\leqslant 7$ ng/g faeces by ELISA, or RPLA titres of 4–8), approaching the limit of detection for the two methods. Retesting these specimens, together with the demonstration of specific neutralization of the toxin, confirmed that, in 13 of the 20 specimens, the variation was not due to false positive or false negative results. In four of the specimens there was insufficient material for retesting and in three (RPLA +, ELISA −) the result of neutralization could not be verified with any confidence and may represent non-specific reactions.

The discrepancy in results that arose with 20 of the specimens is unlikely to be of any practical significance since, with confirmed outbreaks, the majority of faecal specimens collected within 2 days of the onset of symptoms have toxin levels > 1 µg/g (Bartholomew *et al.*, 1985). If, however, specimens are collected 4–6 days after onset, toxin levels are usually low. Nevertheless, even with these outbreaks, some specimens usually have levels of 10–50 ng/g faeces which are readily detected by both methods.

Out of a total of 55 outbreaks investigated, 33 were confirmed as due to *C. perfringens* by the presence of enterotoxin. All 33 were detected by RPLA, with 32 by ELISA. The one equivocal outbreak involved only two people. The faecal specimen of one was negative for enterotoxin by both methods whilst, for the other specimen, the ELISA was negative and the RPLA positive (1:4). Repeat testing of the specimens gave the same result, and the RPLA agglutination reaction was neutralized with anti-enterotoxin.

TABLE 1. *Comparison of the RPLA kit with the plate ELISA for the detection of* C. perfringens *enterotoxin in faeces*

No. of specimens	Enterotoxin detected in faeces by	
	ELISA	RPLA
133	+	+
121	−	−
13	−	+
7	+	−

A disadvantage of the RPLA test is that it is subjective, and occasionally it may be difficult to interpret an agglutination reaction as + (positive) or ± (negative), particularly if there is non-specific agglutination in the control row. Again this problem is unlikely to be of any practical significance, since few specimens (approximately 5%) exhibit non-specific agglutination beyond a dilution of 1:16 (Berry *et al.*, 1986).

In conclusion, the RPLA test is simple, rapid, sensitive, specific and requires no specialized equipment. These conclusions are similar to those of Harmon & Kautter (1986) who evaluated the kit in the U.S.A., using culture supernatants and faecal specimens as test materials. The kit would be of value to routine clinical laboratories, although the cost may be high when considering that a laboratory may not be involved in the investigation of a *C. perfringens* outbreak within the 12 month shelf life of the kit. Many faecal specimens examined routinely are, however, from incidents involving only one or two patients, where no pathogen is detected; a kit such as the RPLA could be used in these circumstances to rule out a *C. perfringens* aetiology, and would give some information on the incidence of *C. perfringens* in small or single-person outbreaks, which we believe are overlooked.

Staphylococcus aureus

Foods from 27 outbreaks were tested for the presence of enterotoxin by the plate ELISA and with the ELISA and RPLA kits, except for four foods which were not tested by the plate ELISA (Table 2: outbreaks 9, 20, 23 and 27), due to insufficient amounts of food sent for testing and the unavailability of reagents for the detection of SEC and SED. Enterotoxin was detected in 20 foods using the ELISA kit and none was found in eight foods, including two combined food samples from outbreaks 25 and 26. A positive and a negative food were obtained from outbreak 18. Results obtained with the two ELISAs always agreed, but of the 20 foods positive with the ELISA kit, three were negative with the RPLA kit and one gave non-specific agglutination (NSA) with the control latex suspension. If a 1:10 food extract had been used as recommended by the manufacturer, enterotoxin would not have been detected in three more foods. When enterotoxin was not detectable by ELISA, the RPLA test was also negative. Except for two foods in which the *S. aureus* had died out, the number of *S. aureus* present in foods in which enterotoxin could be detected was more than 1000 000/g. In enterotoxin negative foods the number of *S. aureus* present was < 1500 000/g.

Twenty samples of food, including fish, meat and their products, cheese and pasta, which were not connected with staphylococcal food poisoning were examined for the presence of enterotoxin with the two kits. *S. aureus* was not found in 10 of these foods and the remaining 10 foods contained only low numbers of an enterotoxigenic strain. Enterotoxin was not detected in any of the foods. Two extracts of sheep milk cheese showed NSA with the control latex suspension.

TABLE 2. *Detection of enterotoxin in foods from outbreaks of staphylococcal food poisoning by three different methods*

Outbreak number	Food	Count of S. aureus/g	Enterotoxin produced by strain	Enterotoxin detected in food by		
				plate ELISA	ELISA kit	RPLA kit
1	Ham	1.5×10^9	A	+	+	+
2	Vanilla slice	1.3×10^9	A	+	+	+
3	Ham	9.0×10^8	A	+	+	+
4	Turkey and duck	3.0×10^8	A	+	+	+
5	Lasagne—dried	2.0×10^8	A	+	+	+
6	Roast beef	1.0×10^8	A	+	+	+
7	Corned beef	1.5×10^7	A	+	+	+
8	Salmon canned	3.5×10^6	A	+	+	+
9	Ham	3.0×10^6	A	NT	+	−
10	Halloumi cheese	ND		+	+	+
11	Sheep's milk cheese	ND		+	+	NSA
12	Corned beef	4.5×10^7	AB	+[b]	+[d]	+[d]
13	Corned beef	4.0×10^7	AB	+	+	+
14	Ham	1.2×10^9	AD	+[c]	+	+[c]
15	Smokey bacon spread	1.0×10^9	AD	+[c]	+	+
16	Salmon—mousse	9.0×10^8	AD	+[c]	+	+[c]
17	Ham rolls	5.0×10^8	AD	+[c]	+	+[c]
18	Beef rolls	4.0×10^6	AD	+[c]	+[e]	−[c]
19	Pork	6.0×10^9	B	+	+	+
20	Chicken	1.0×10^6	C	NT	+	−
21	Chicken chow mein	1.5×10^6	A	−	−	−
22	Meat pies	1.0×10^6	A	−	−	−
23	Ham	5.0×10^5	A	NT	−	−
24	Corned beef	8.5×10^4	A	−	−	−
25[a]	Cold buffet	$\leqslant 700$	A	−	−	−
26[a]	Cold buffet	6.0×10^3	AB	−	−	−
18	Sausage rolls	2.0×10^4	AD	−[c]	−	−
27	Meat lasagne dish	5.0×10^4	D	NT	−	−

ND = not detected. NT = not tested. NSA = non specific agglutination. a = several different foods tested. b = extract not tested for SEB. c = extract not tested for SED. d = SEB was not detected. e = SED was not detected.

The manufacturer's instructions supplied with the ELISA kit state that the factors obtained by dividing the absorbance value at 405 nm of the sample by $\bar{x} + 3 \times$ standard deviation (where $\bar{x}$ is the mean absorbance value obtained with the NRS-IgG coated beads) is normally 5–20 for positive foods. In this study the calculated factor was > 5 for all positive foods.

The absorbance values with the control beads usually ranged from 0–0.02

except in tests for SED where values as high as 0.45 were occasionally obtained, in which case positive results might be obscured.

When NSA occurs with the control latex of the RPLA kit, the test can still be interpreted as positive when agglutination with sensitized latex occurs with a higher dilution of the test sample than that with the latex control. In this study, this effect was found once with the sample of lasagne. Enterotoxins found in food extracts with the RPLA test were all neutralized by 0.1% homologous antiserum.

TABLE 3.   *Comparison of methods*

	C. perfringens enterotoxin		Staphylococcal enterotoxin		
	RPLA	plate ELISA	RPLA	plate ELISA	Kit ELISA
Cost per test (materials)	£2.50	~20p	£5.00	~50p	£6.00
Time required for completion of test (time for extraction excluded)	24 h	8 h	24 h	8 h	24 h
Labour intensity of extraction	Low	Low	Low/high	High	High
Labour intensity of test	Low	Moderate	Low	Moderate	High
Sensitivity (ng/g)	2–4	2–4	4–40	2	0.1–1
Specificity	Good/ excellent	Excellent	Good	Excellent	Good/ excellent
Subjectivity	Yes	No	Yes	No	No
Specialized equipment	No	Yes	No	Yes	Yes

A summary of the performance of the three methods is given in Table 3. The ELISA kit was the most sensitive method, although, with the SED reagents a high blank occasionally obscured the results. Also the test was fairly laborious. The RPLA test was easy to carry out, but its sensitivity was insufficient to detect enterotoxin in all foods that were positive with the ELISA kit. Also NSA might obscure positive results. Neither kit contained reagents for the detection of SEE, because of its infrequent occurrence. Used side by side, the two kits complement each other.

Acknowledgements

We are grateful to the Public Health Laboratory Service and hospital laboratories who sent us samples of foods or faecal specimens from outbreaks of food poisoning, and to our colleague Dr Diane Roberts for her help in producing this paper.

References

BARTHOLOMEW, B. A., STRINGER, M. F., WATSON, G. N. & GILBERT, R. J. 1985 Development and application of an enzyme-linked immunosorbent assay for *Clostridium perfringens* type A enterotoxin. *Journal of Clinical Pathology* 38, 222–228.

BERRY, P. R., STRINGER, M. F. & UEMURA, T. 1986 Comparison of latex agglutination and ELISA for the detection of *Clostridium perfringens* type A enterotoxin in faeces. *Letters in Applied Microbiology* 2, 101–102.

FEY, H., PFISTER, H. & RÜGG, O. 1984 Comparative evaluation of different enzyme-linked immunosorbent assay systems for the detection of staphylococcal enterotoxins A, B, C and D. *Journal of Clinical Microbiology* 19, 34–38.

GILBERT, R. J., WIENEKE, A. A., LANSER, J. & ŠIMKOVOČOVÁ, M. 1972 Serological detection of enterotoxin in foods implicated in staphylococcal food poisoning. *Journal of Hygiene* 70, 755–762.

HARMON, S. M. & KAUTTER, D. A. 1986 Evaluation of a reversed passive latex agglutination test kit for *Clostridium perfringens* enterotoxin. *Journal of Food Protection* 49, 523–525.

HOBBS, B. C., SMITH, M. E., OAKLEY, C. L., WARRACK, G. H. & CRUICKSHANK, J. C. 1953 *Clostridium welchii* food poisoning. *Journal of Hygiene* 51, 75–101.

IGARASHI, H., SHINGAKI, M., FUJIKAWA, H., USHIODA, H. & TERAYAMA, T. 1985 Detection of staphylococcal enterotoxins in food poisoning outbreaks by reversed passive latex agglutination. In *The Staphylococci Proceedings of the Vth International Symposium on Staphylococci and Staphylococcal Infections* Warsaw 26–30 June 1984 ed. Jeljaszewicz, J. pp. 255–257. Stuttgart: Gustave Fischer Verlag.

NOTERMANS, S., BOOT, R., TIPS, P. D. & DE NOOY, M. P. 1983 Extraction of staphylococcal enterotoxins (SE) from minced meat and subsequent detection of SE with enzyme-linked immunosorbent assay (ELISA). *Journal of Food Protection* 46, 238–241.

REISER, R., CONAWAY, D. & BERGDOLL, M. S. 1974 Detection of staphylococcal enterotoxin in foods. *Applied Microbiology* 27, 83–85.

SHINGAKI, S., IGARASHI, H., FUJIKAWA, H., USHIODA, H., TERAYAMA, T. & SAKAI, S. 1981 Study on reversed passive latex agglutination for the detection of staphylococcal enterotoxins A–C. *Annual Report of the Tokyo Metropolitan Research Laboratory of Public Health* 32, 128–131.

STRINGER, M. F. 1985 *Clostridium perfringens* type A food poisoning. In *Clostridia in Gastrointestinal Disease* ed. Borriello, S. P. pp. 117–143. London: CRC Press.

STRINGER, M. F., WATSON, G. N. & GILBERT, R. J. 1982 *Clostridium perfringens* type A: serological typing and methods for the detection of enterotoxin. In *Isolation and Identification Methods for Food Poisoning Organisms*, SAB Technical Series No. 17 ed. Corry, J. E. L., Roberts, D. & Skinner, F. A. pp. 111–135. London: Academic Press.

STRINGER, M. F., WATSON, G. N., GILBERT, R. J., WALLACE, J. G., HASSALL, J. E., TANNER, E. I. & WEBBER, P. P. 1985 Faecal carriage of *Clostridium perfringens*. *Journal of Hygiene* 95, 277–288.

SUTTON, R. G. A. & HOBBS, B. C. 1968 Food poisoning caused by heat-sensitive *Clostridium welchii*. A report of five recent outbreaks. *Journal of Hygiene* 66, 135–146.

WIENEKE, A. A. & GILBERT, R. J. 1985 The use of a sandwich ELISA for the detection of staphylococcal enterotoxin A in foods from outbreaks of food poisoning. *Journal of Hygiene* 95, 131–138.

WIENEKE, A. A. & GILBERT, R. J. 1987 Comparison of four methods for the detection of staphylococcal enterotoxin in foods from outbreaks of food poisoning. *International Journal of Food Microbiology* 4, 135–143.

WIMSATT, J. C., HARMON, S. M. & SHAH, D. B. 1986 Detection of *Clostridium perfringens* in stool specimens and culture supernatants by enzyme linked immunosorbent assay. *Diagnostic Microbiology and Infectious Disease* 4, 307–313.

Meat Species Identification: a Semi-Quantitative ELISA-based Test to Confirm the Species of a Given Meat and to Detect Contamination of one Meat Species with Another*

JANE PELLY AND R. W. TINDLE

Sera-Lab Ltd, Crawley Down, West Sussex RH10 4FF

Introduction

The meat species identification test is a simple and rapid test procedure based on enzyme immunoassay (ELISA). It has been designed to confirm the species of the meat sample and to detect contamination of one meat species with another at levels of $> 1\%$ w/w. It is intended for use with uncooked meats.

Principle of Technique

The assay employs the 'sandwich system'. Anti-meat protein antibody is adsorbed to the wells of a PVC microtitre tray and the meat extract under test added. Bound antigen is visualized by using urease conjugated species specific antibody.

Kit contents

Solution 1:   wash buffer $10 \times$ concentrated.
Solution 2:   urease conjugated species specific anti-meat protein antibody.
Solution 3:   urease substrate solution (sterile).
Reaction tray: a 96 well PVC tray to which anti-meat protein antibody has been adsorbed.
Sealing tapes: for sealing trays during incubation stages.

Method

Each test must include a set of control samples. These may be prepared by diluting extracts from authenticated meat samples to appropriate levels e.g. 100%, 10%,

---

* This test has been developed by Commonwealth Serum Laboratories (Australia) and is marketed by Sera-Lab Ltd, Crawley Down, West Sussex.

Immunological Techniques
in Microbiology

1% and 0% in washing buffer. Control solutions should be prepared for each species being tested.

1 Prepare an extract of the meat sample under test by adding 1.5 ml of distilled water/g of meat and vigorously shaking and mixing for 1 min. Leave the mixture for 10 min at room temperature to allow the solid residue to settle before drawing off an aliquot for testing. To prepare the 100% extract add one part of solution 1, to nine parts of aqueous meat extract.

2 The PVC tray may be cut to supply the required number of wells and the rest stored for further use. Remove the sealing tape from the tray and discard the contents of the wells. Wash the tray section three times in diluted wash buffer taking care to empty the wells between each wash. Wipe any excess moisture from the top of the tray section with a tissue.

3 Add 100 µl of the appropriate test and control samples to separate wells, reseal the tray and incubate at 37 °C for 30 min.

4 Carefully remove the sealing tape avoiding contamination of samples in adjacent wells, and remove the samples, preferably by vacuum aspiration.

5 Wash the tray section three times with diluted wash buffer and add 100 µl of solution 2 to each well, reseal and incubate for 30 min at 37 °C.

6 Discard the contents of the wells and wash the tray section a further three times with diluted wash buffer and then three times with distilled water.

7 Add 100 µl of solution 3 to each well and allow to stand at room temperature, observing the tray at intervals over the next 30 min. Record the results when the solution in the well of the 1% control meat sample has changed to a definite purple colour. If, after observation for 30 min the 1% control sample has not changed to definite purple the test is invalid.

Interpretation of results

Species confirmation

A positive result is indicated by a colour change from yellow to purple in the test well.

Species contamination

Contamination is indicated by a positive result on a heterologous plate. The level of contamination may be estimated by comparison with the intensity and rate of colour change observed with the control sample wells.

Advantages of the Urease Method

The enzymes most frequently used to label the tracer reagent in ELISA procedures are horseradish peroxidase and alkaline phosphatase, but for a rapid field type assay kit these enzymes have disadvantages. Both use substrates which are unstable in aqueous solution, making it necessary to prepare fresh solutions just prior to use, and neither has substrates which give an easily recognized colour change.

Commonwealth Serum Laboratories have introduced the enzyme urease and a substrate solution consisting of urea and the pH indicator bromocresol purple (Chandler *et al.*, 1982). Urease gives a highly visual colour change (yellow to purple) with sharp endpoint when used with the stable urea-indicator substrate solution, making it particularly useful for mass screening and field type ELISA procedures. Urease has the added advantage that it does not occur in mammalian tissues, and this makes it highly suitable for use in tests for cell-associated antigens. Finally, the enzyme reaction may be stopped by addition of organomercurial preservatives, allowing storage of tests for later examination.

Appendix: Kits Currently Available

Beef Species Identification Test
Horse Species Identification Test
Kangaroo Species Identification Test
Sheep Species Identification Test
Goat Species Identification Test
Pig Species Identification Test
Camel Species Identification Test
Buffalo Species Identification Test
Donkey Species Identification Test

Reference

CHANDLER, H. M., COX, J. C., HEALEY, K., MacGREGOR, A., PREMIER, R. R. & HURRELL, J. G. R. 1982 An investigation of the use of urease-antibody conjugates in enzyme immunoassays. *Journal of Immunological Methods* 53, 187–194.

Commercial and 'In-House' Assays—a Comparison Exemplified by Assays for Antibodies to the AIDS Virus

R. J. S. DUNCAN

Wellcome Diagnostics, Langley Court, Beckenham, Kent BR3 3BS

Introduction: Development of a Commercial Assay

The development of the current Wellcozyme™ *anti*-HTLV-III (*anti*-HIV) test will be used as an example of collaboration between industrial and academic laboratories to meet the demand for an assay for a particular virus. The major point to be made is that there are two aspects of a commercial diagnostic kit, first the assay itself and second the 'peripheral' things such as quality assurance, equipment, training and packaging. Devising the assay method is often only a comparatively minor and less demanding part of the work involved in developing a satisfactory product and more time is often spent in ensuring 'robustness', ease of use, and reproducibility than on the assay system itself.

Differences Between Commercial and Laboratory Assays

The primary differences between a laboratory test and a commercially useful diagnostic test are a result of differences in the experience and training of the users. A laboratory test is operated by a highly trained and motivated user, often the originator of the system, who can make decisions about the results that he gets in the light of experience of both the assay and the samples tested. The commercial test, on the other hand, may well be used by a far less well trained person, and it is necessary that the assay works reliably, and can be shown to have worked reliably, even in inexperienced hands. For this reason, the commercial test will have undergone extensive testing with difficult and uncommon samples which the designer of a laboratory test could expect to consider individually as they arose, and the behaviour of the commercial test with those samples will be fully documented. Similarly, the commercial test will give a very clear cut distinction between positive and negative samples so that discrimination is easy even to an untrained user, and there will be internal quality control parameters so that the user knows that the

Immunological Techniques
in Microbiology

assay has performed adequately even though he may not understand the principles of the system. The design of a commercial assay is of importance in assuring the quality of the results: all pipettings and dilutions must be very easy to do correctly, and the accuracy of the assay is usually made as independent as possible of the exact volumes of the reagents. A commercial assay must also be designed so that it fits smoothly into the routine of the laboratories in which it is intended to be used—presenting fewer chances for the user to make errors. Esoteric or highly accurate apparatus is not normally required for commercial kits because, for wide acceptability, they must operate in routine laboratories where equipment may be at a premium: this relates to the requirement that a commercial assay gives good discrimination between positive and negative samples. While the manufacturer will often supply apparatus, it is not a commercial proposition to provide dedicated apparatus to all possible users especially if the apparatus is not already widely available. From this it will be clear that for commercial applicability it is not sufficient merely for an assay to work well. That is the simple aspect and is taken for granted. Additionally a commercial assay must be robust and essentially foolproof.

So far the assay itself has been considered, but other aspects also assume importance because a commercial assay will be used by inexperienced operators in busy laboratories. Stability of the components of a kit is crucial, not only to ensure a long shelf life of the system, but also so that an inexperienced user cannot waste valuable reagents by poor storage conditions and so that the assay can be used in non-ideal environments. Also, the dangers of the reagents used in the commercial format is of concern. While a scientist may be able to use hazardous chemicals or microbiological procedures in safety in a research laboratory, commercial kits must be usable by non-experts in complete safety in routine laboratories.

There is a large difference in the scale of operation between laboratory and commercial assays, for example approximately 25 000 AIDS tests are performed each working day in the U.K. alone. Fortunately it is not difficult to scale up the preparation of diagnostic kits so long as the physical plant (microbiological containment facilities, freeze-driers, tableting machines, packing lines) is available; the difficulties are related to ensuring the quality control of the finished and part finished product, and in efficient production control to integrate the manufacture of different kits which are made on the same plant.

Laboratory and Commercial HIV Assays

Our collaborators at the Middlesex Hospital Medical School and the Chester Beatty Laboratories provided us with reagents and methods for a radioimmunoassay for antibodies to the HIV. It was clear that the format they suggested—a competitive ('inhibition') assay using immobilized HIV antigens—was excellent but that the details of the assay required optimization for direct commercial use. Although the assay worked well in a research laboratory environment the distinction between positive and negative samples was unsatisfactory in the hands of inexpert users and the sample-to-sample variation was too great. The presentation of the solid phase was also unsatisfactory, and illustrates a difference between a useful laboratory tactic and commercial requirements. Microtitre plates for the radioassay were stored under liquid in the cold, while for the commercial kit it was necessary to present the plates in a very stable dry form. Radioimmunoassay is now perceived as out-dated technology and cannot be sold in several important export markets, so the underlying detection system of the assay had to be changed. These changes—separating the signals from positive and negative samples, lowering the coefficient of variation of the test, stabilizing the plates by an economic method, and converting the whole system to an enzyme immunoassay—involved an intensive effort to harness and adapt the technology existing within Wellcome Diagnostics. At the same time our in-house skills of freeze-drying, conjugate preparation and stabilization, plate coating and washing, and enzyme detection were all employed. Collaboration with the Microbiology Department at the Public Health Laboratories at Porton ensured a reliable supply of the viral antigens on a commercial scale after a considerable effort had been made there to devise methods of growing and inactivating the virus in large amounts.

At that stage it could be seen that the kit would work well, as expected, and it was necessary to undertake the 'peripheral' activities of converting the laboratory assay into its final commercial form and to begin the large investment required for the successful manufacture of any product.

A wide range of difficult and unusual samples was tested, as well as many thousands of normal blood donations. The stability of typical production batches of the kit was measured, and the methods of stabilizing the conjugate and plates were finalized so that the Good Manufacturing Practice requirement of 28 days stability at 37 °C could be achieved. It then was possible to set up both in-assay and in-manufacture quality control criteria, and to document the behaviour of the system. Quality control of the kit (including quality assurance input during the format design stages) has historically involved more people and more time than the development of the assay itself and is a commitment throughout the life of the product.

Marketing decisions about the number of tests per kit and the type and detail of packaging had to be made, labels printed, and the user instructions written in the required format. Whilst this was being done, the production and packing teams were being trained in the routines of manufacturing the kit, and the final production protocols were written. Decisions about the level and type of equipment and computing support to supply with the kit were taken, and instruments were purchased on a forecast of demand. Throughout, the sales force had to be kept fully informed of the progress on the system, and the representatives were trained in the background science of both AIDS and ELISA, how to use the kit, how to teach others to use the kit, and basic error elimination in the user's laboratories.

The successful commercial presentation of what is already a good, working laboratory assay requires a large amount of skill and capital investment; also an understanding of the problems and requirements faced by industry smoothes the early stages of collaboration between the originators of a test and the potential manufacturers.

Index

263

THE SOCIETY FOR APPLIED BACTERIOLOGY TECHNICAL SERIES

General Editor: F. A. Skinner